DENVER PUBLIC SCHOOLS

3 7137 04809271 9   613.7 ROZ
Core training

D1791847

FITNESS AND TRAINING

CORE TRAINING

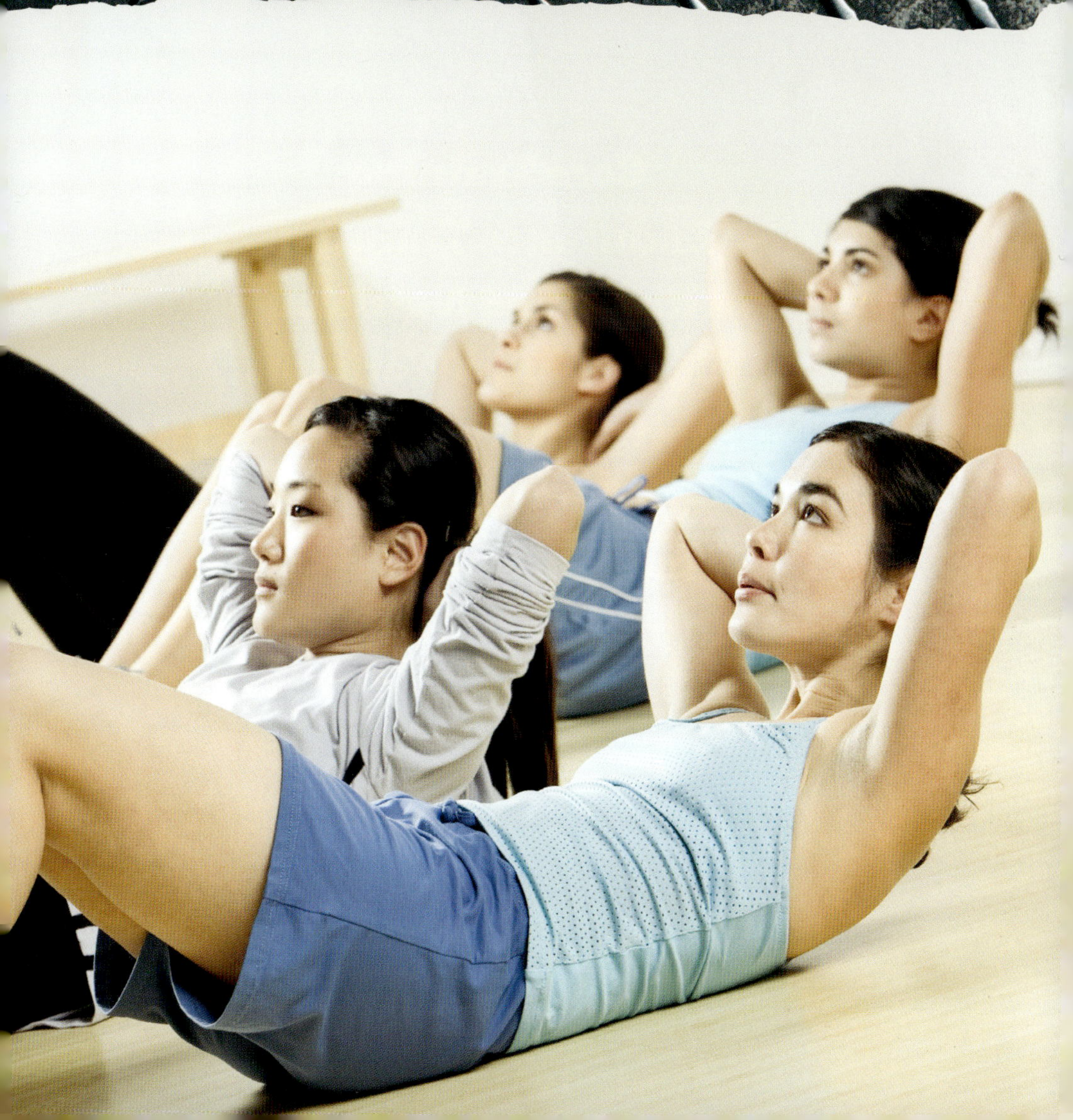

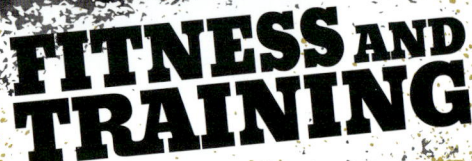

FITNESS AND TRAINING

Core Training
Endurance Training
Fitness and Nutrition
High-Energy Workouts
High-Intensity Interval Training (HIIT)
Low Impact Training
Mind and Body Fitness
Strength and Bodyweight Training

FITNESS AND TRAINING
CORE TRAINING

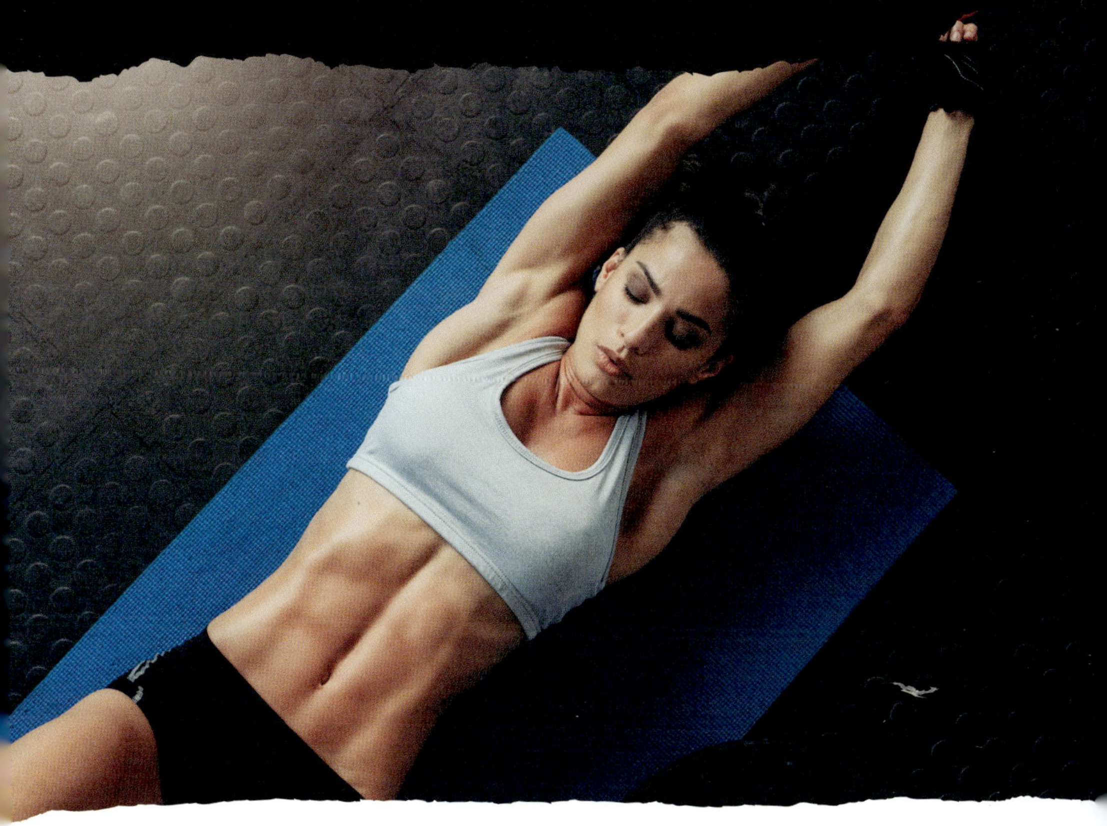

Kimber Rozier

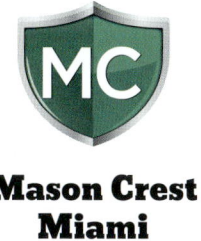

Mason Crest
Miami

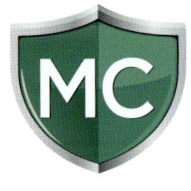

Mason Crest
PO Box 221876
Hollywood, FL 33022
(866) MCP-BOOK (toll-free)
www.masoncrest.com

Copyright © 2023 by Mason Crest, an imprint of National Highlights, Inc. All rights reserved. No part of this publication may be reproduced or transmitted in any form or by any means, electronic or mechanical, including photocopying, recording, taping, or any information storage and retrieval system, without permission from the publisher.

First printing
9 8 7 6 5 4 3 2 1
ISBN (hardback) 978-1-4222-4595-8
ISBN (series) 978-1-4222-4594-1
ISBN (ebook) 978-1-4222-7211-4

Library of Congress Cataloging-in-Publication Data

Names: Rozier, Kimber, author.
Title: Core training / Kimber Rozier.
Description: Hollywood, FL : Mason Crest, 2023. | Series: Fitness and training | Includes bibliographical references and index.
Identifiers: LCCN 2020003354 | ISBN 9781422245958 (hardback) | ISBN 9781422272114 (ebook)
Subjects: LCSH: Abdominal exercises–Juvenile literature. | Abdomen–Muscles–Juvenile literature. | Physical fitness–Juvenile literature. | Muscle strength–Juvenile literature.
Classification: LCC GV508 .R69 2021 | DDC 613.7/1886–dc23
LC record available at https://lccn.loc.gov/2020003354

Developed and Produced by National Highlights, Inc.
Editor: Andrew Luke
Production: Crafted Content, LLC

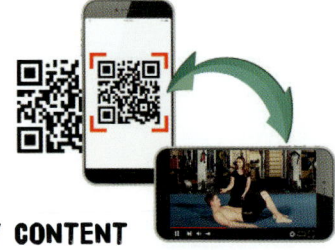

QR CODES AND LINKS TO THIRD-PARTY CONTENT

You may gain access to certain third-party content ("Third-Party Sites") by scanning and using the QR Codes that appear in this publication (the "QR Codes"). We do not operate or control in any respect any information, products, or services on such Third-Party Sites linked to by us via the QR Codes included in this publication, and we assume no responsibility for any materials you may access using the QR Codes. Your use of the QR Codes may be subject to terms, limitations, or restrictions set forth in the applicable terms of use or otherwise established by the owners of the Third-Party Sites. Our linking to such Third-Party Sites via the QR Codes does not imply an endorsement or sponsorship of such Third-Party Sites or the information, products, or services offered on or through the Third-Party Sites, nor does it imply an endorsement or sponsorship of this publication by the owners of such Third-Party Sites.

CONTENTS

Chapter 1: Core Training: What it is and Why it Helps 7
Chapter 2: Core Anatomy and Biomechanics 17
Chapter 3: Assessing the Core: Strength vs. Stability 29
Chapter 4: The Science of Core Stability 43
Chapter 5: Sport-Specific Core Training 53
Chapter 6: Common Injuries: How Core Training
           Prevents Them. 65
Chapter 7: Core Training Exercises 77
Series Glossary of Key Terms 92
Further Reading & Internet Resources 93
Index 94
Author Biography, Photo Credits & Educational Video Links . . 96

KEY ICONS TO LOOK FOR

WORDS TO UNDERSTAND: These words, with their easy-to-understand definitions, will increase readers' understanding of the text while building vocabulary skills.

SIDEBARS: This boxed material within the main text allows readers to build knowledge, gain insights, explore possibilities, and broaden their perspectives by weaving together additional information to provide realistic and holistic perspectives.

EDUCATIONAL VIDEOS: Readers can view videos by scanning our QR codes, providing them with additional educational content to supplement the text.

TEXT-DEPENDENT QUESTIONS: These questions send the reader back to the text for more careful attention to the evidence presented there.

RESEARCH PROJECTS: Readers are pointed toward areas of further inquiry connected to each chapter. Suggestions are provided for projects that encourage deeper research and analysis.

SERIES GLOSSARY OF KEY TERMS: This back-of-the-book glossary contains terminology used throughout this series. Words found here increase the reader's ability to read and comprehend higher-level books and articles in this field.

WORDS TO UNDERSTAND

global systems—muscles that run from the pelvis to the thoracic cage to help transfer energy between the lower and upper body

kinetic chain—a group of interconnected joints and muscles that work together to perform a task

local systems—muscles of the core with insertions or origins along the lumbar spine which help generate stiffness

pelvic floor—a group of muscles at the base of the pelvis supporting the organs

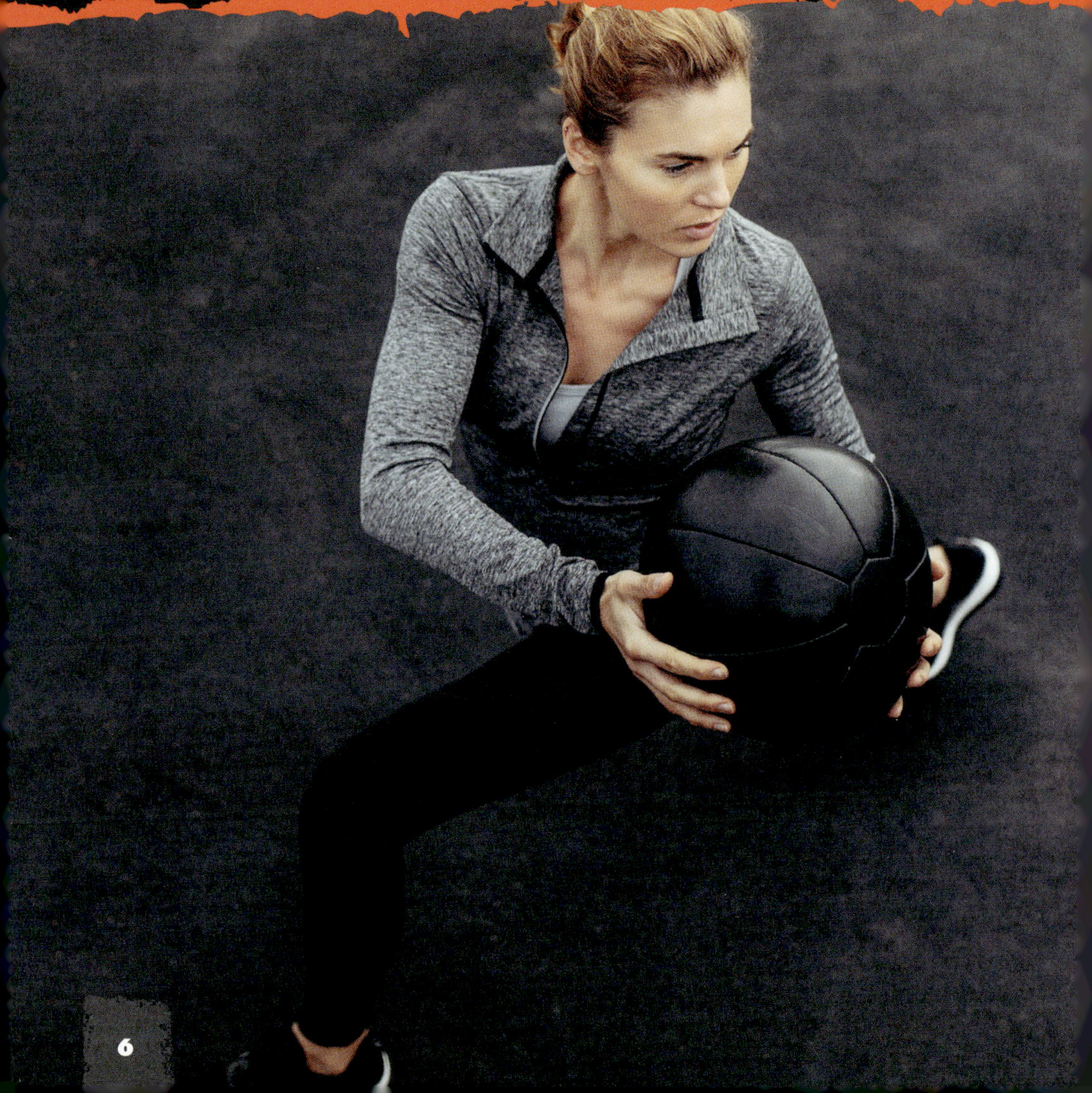

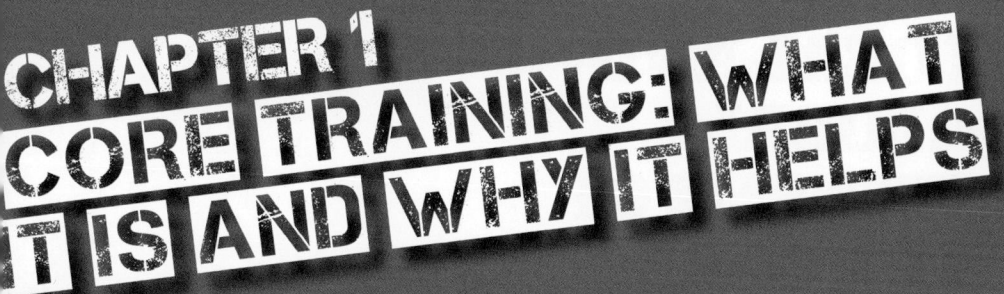

CHAPTER 1
CORE TRAINING: WHAT IT IS AND WHY IT HELPS

If you want to move well, become strong, and retain a balanced physique, you need to train the core. As such, people toss around the term "core training" for all types of workouts. But what does it truly involve? In this chapter, we'll answer that question and more, illuminating the benefits of training this critical section of the body.

HOW DO YOU DEFINE THE CORE?

Even the scientific community has trouble answering this question. Everyone agrees that your core includes the midsection, somewhere around your abdominals, hips, and lower back. But many disagree on the exact muscles that qualify. For example, the core has been described as a cylinder between the diaphragm and **pelvic floor,** including those muscles, the abdominals (abs), the gluteus maximus, medius and minimus (glutes), and erector spinae (paraspinals). Other experts want to include the latissimus dorsi (lats), rhomboids, pectorals (pecs), and other muscles that connect the shoulders to the spine. Some even argue that your core continues all the way to the knees.

Your core protects the spine and stabilizes the rest of the body throughout movement. Therefore, it helps control the limbs, pelvis, rib cage, and even the head and neck. It's such a critical piece of the **kinetic chain** that, theoretically, multiple muscles fit the bill. To help illuminate their function, we can categorize the muscles into **local and global systems.**

LOCAL AND GLOBAL SYSTEMS OF THE CORE

Local muscles have insertions or origins along the lumbar spine and provide stiffness for spinal stability. For example, the muscles of the erector spinae lie just along either side of the spine to provide protection during any potentially dangerous movement or activity. Moreover, the transverse abdominis (TVA) acts like a corset wrapped around the midsection, locking everything into place.

In contrast, the global muscles run from the pelvis to the thoracic cage and therefore help transfer energy between the lower and upper body. These muscles, such as the rectus abdominis and obliques, allow for healthy movement. Core function relies on a balance and coordination of the strength and stability of these two systems.

For the purposes of this book, we're going to focus on the double-sided cylinder between the diaphragm and pelvic floor, including the glutes, abs, and lower back musculature.

WHY IS THE CORE SO DIFFICULT TO IDENTIFY?

If we think about the function of the core, it becomes easier to understand. In English, the word "core" refers to a central part of something, usually lying deep within. Just think of the Earth's core, the core of an argument, or the core of an apple. Therefore, everyone agrees that when referring to the body, the core relates to the spine while stationary. It's when movement gets involved that things become tricky. What muscles lie at the center of every movement? Do we include the nerves, bones, connective tissue, and organs? It's a tough question to answer, and we continue to wait for the scientific community to come to a consensus.

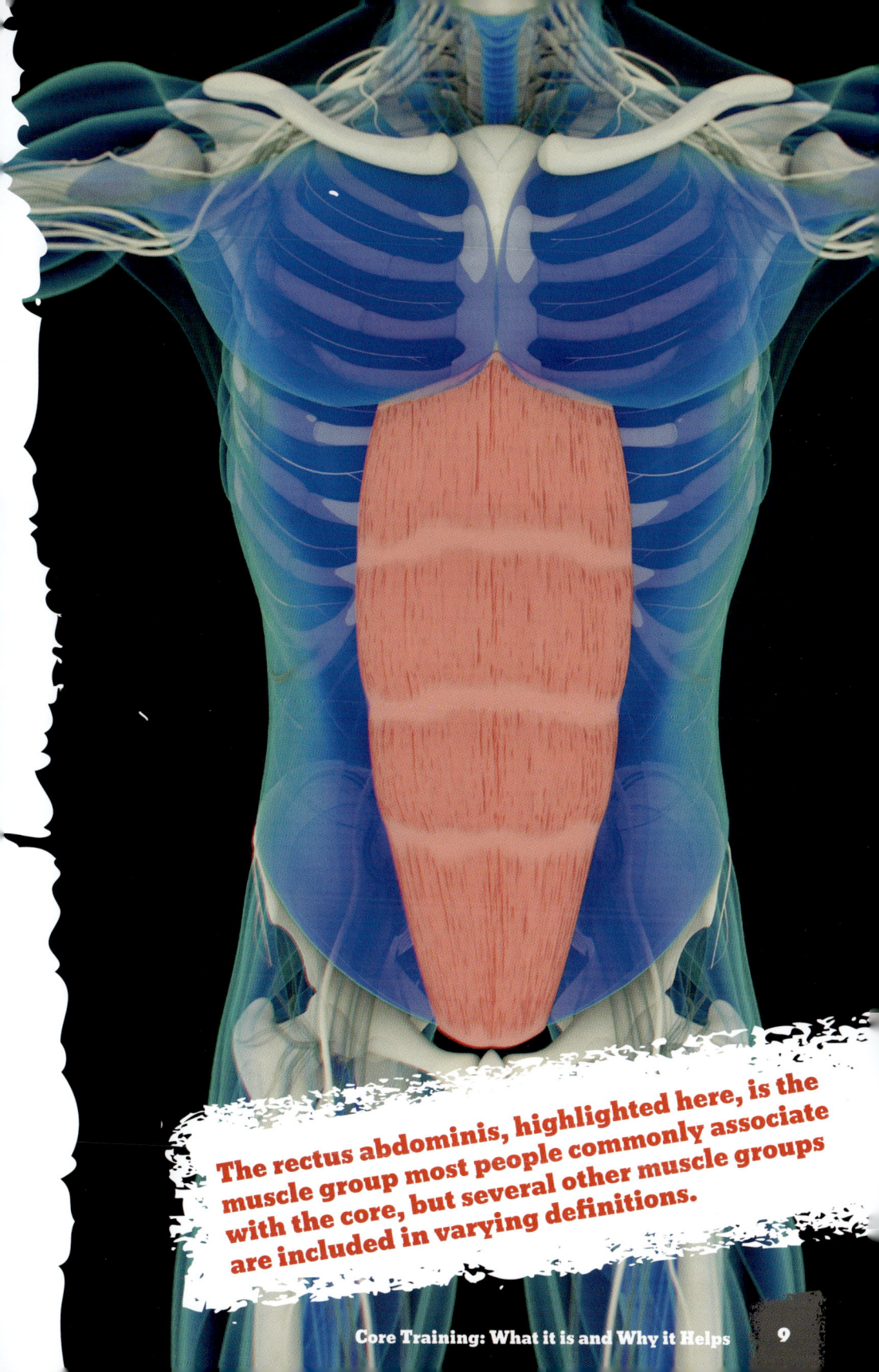

The rectus abdominis, highlighted here, is the muscle group most people commonly associate with the core, but several other muscle groups are included in varying definitions.

 What is core training? Watch this for an answer.

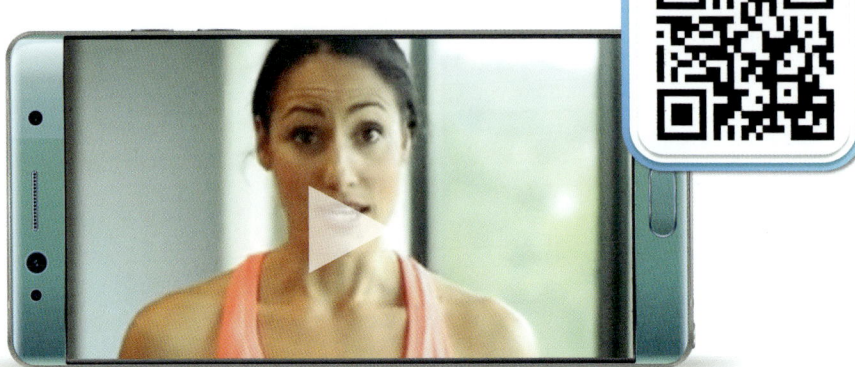

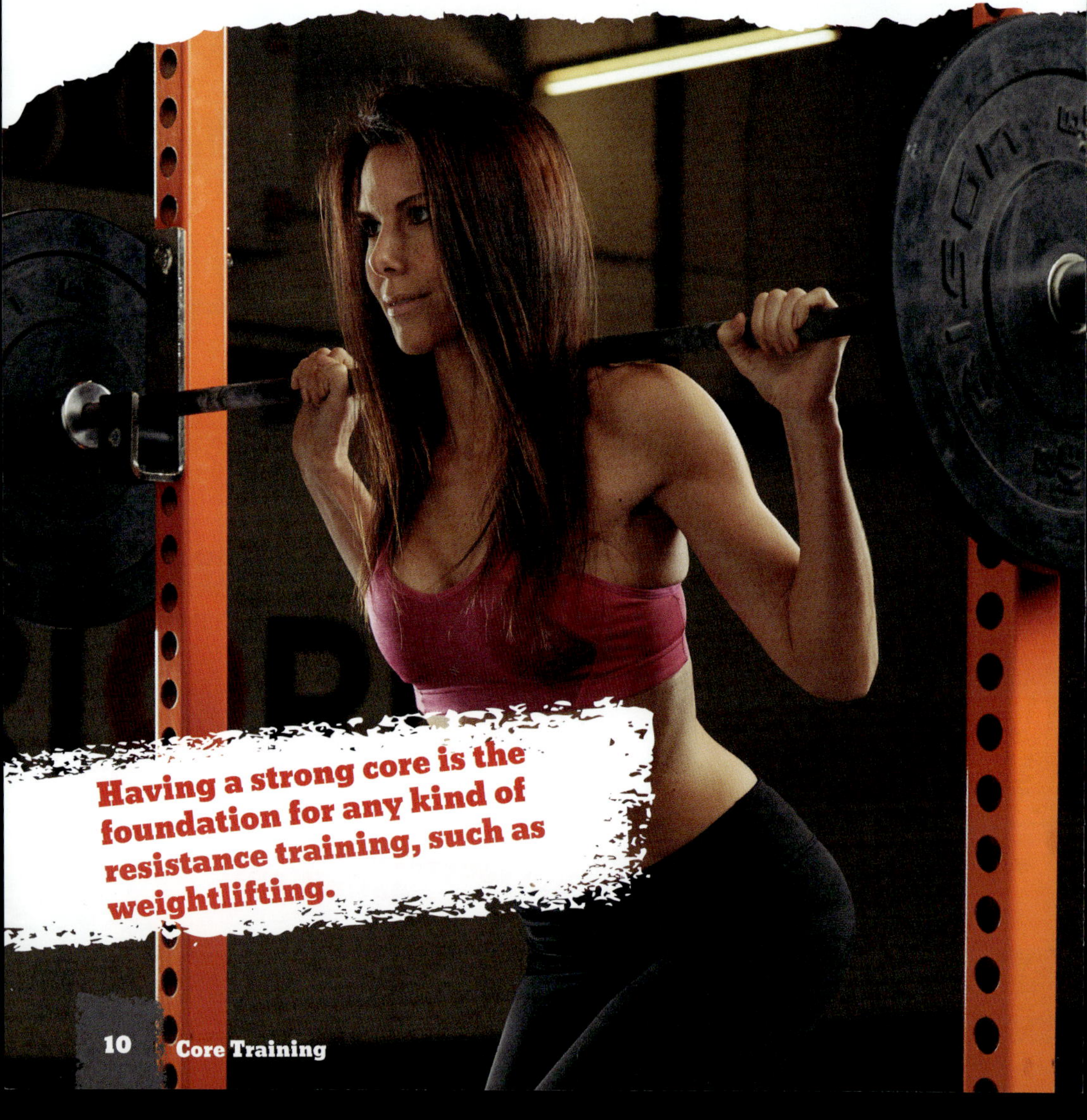

Having a strong core is the foundation for any kind of resistance training, such as weightlifting.

WHAT ARE THE BENEFITS OF CORE TRAINING?

In the fitness world, core training has become synonymous with athletic performance and injury prevention; therefore having a strong, stable core keeps you healthy. Of course, there's always the appearance question. Even if the coveted "six-pack" drives a lot of abdominal workouts, we can't ignore all of the other benefits of core training.

Better Workouts

Given the role of the core in energy transfer, having a strong core enhances your workout as a whole. Any kind of resistance training, whether bodyweight or weightlifting, relies on the core as a foundation. It helps you control the bar in a squat, transfers speed and power in ballistic movements, and keeps you moving during cardio sessions.

Research shows that your core muscles activate in preparation for movement. The TVA controls lumbar movement by contracting slightly before lower limb activity. As local stability of the spine correlates with global power transfer, with a strong core you could lift more weight or run faster before fatigue or injury occurs. More effective workouts lead to quicker results. In addition, if you can avoid injury, you can stay consistent in the gym.

Athletic Performance

It's widely accepted that improved core strength and stability lead to improved athletic performance. We know that the core directly controls hip function for activities like jumping, cutting, throwing, and squatting. It also makes sense that a strong foundation leads to strength and ability further down the chain. As the saying goes, it's hard to shoot a cannon out of a canoe. In theory, the core affects athletic performance through trunk stabilization during technical movements. It also helps transfer force from the lower to the upper body and directly controls rotational athletic movements.

Unfortunately, it's difficult to isolate these results in the lab, as so many factors are at play. Therefore, according to research, the results are mixed on the effect of core strengthening on athletic performance. According to the journal *Sports Medicine,* the lack of gold standard measurements of strength, along with the high-load, resisted, dynamic nature of athletic movement make definitive claims difficult.

Some studies do show a correlation between improvements in core strength and stability and athletic performance. Athletes with greater core strength exhibit higher squat and bench press numbers, faster rotational swings, and better 40-yard dash times. Other studies found a weak, inconsistent correlation between core stability and the vertical jump, shuttle run, 20/40-yard sprints, and 1-rep max lift performance.

Research shows that athletes with greater core strength performed better in several exercises, including the bench press.

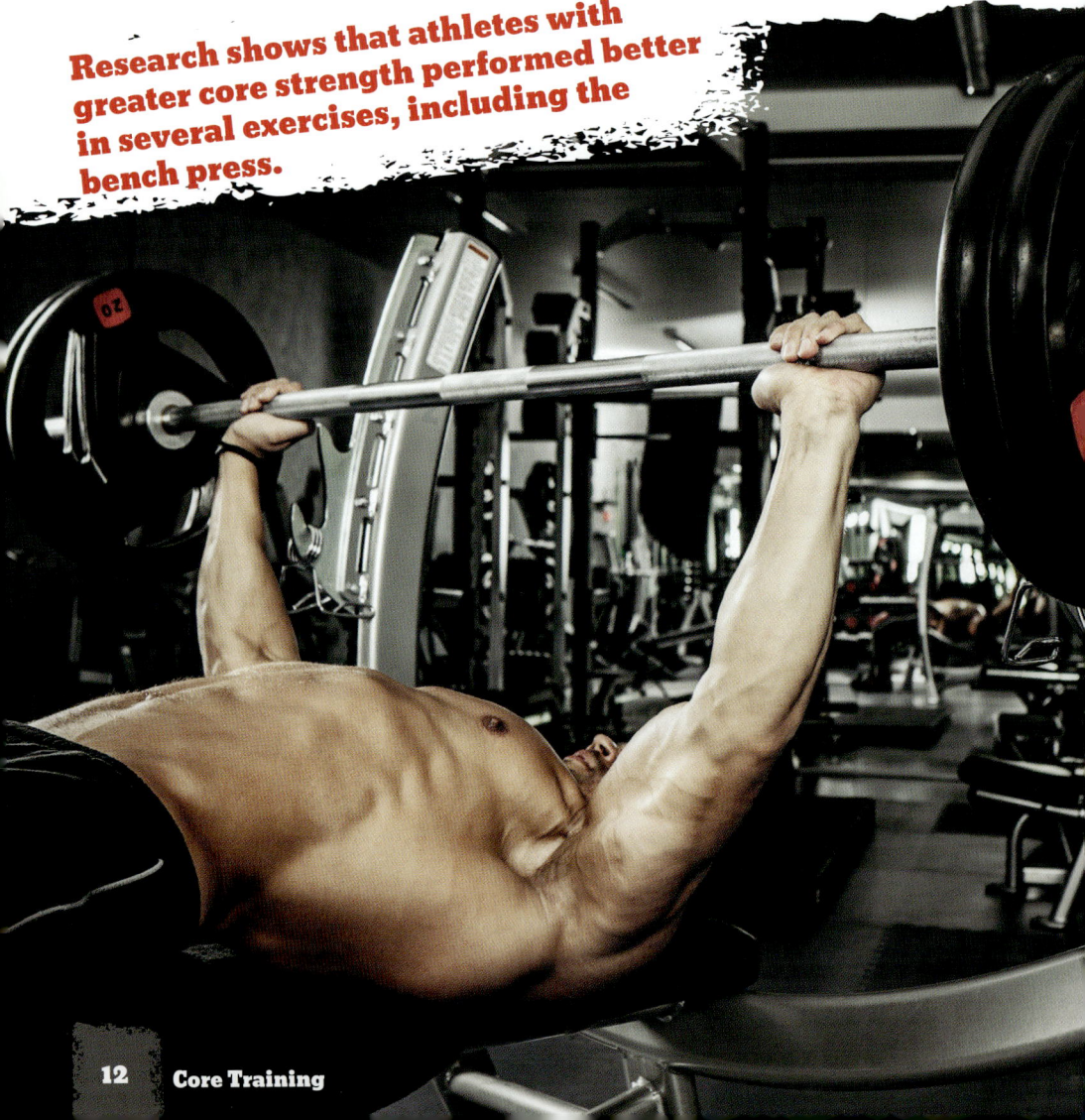

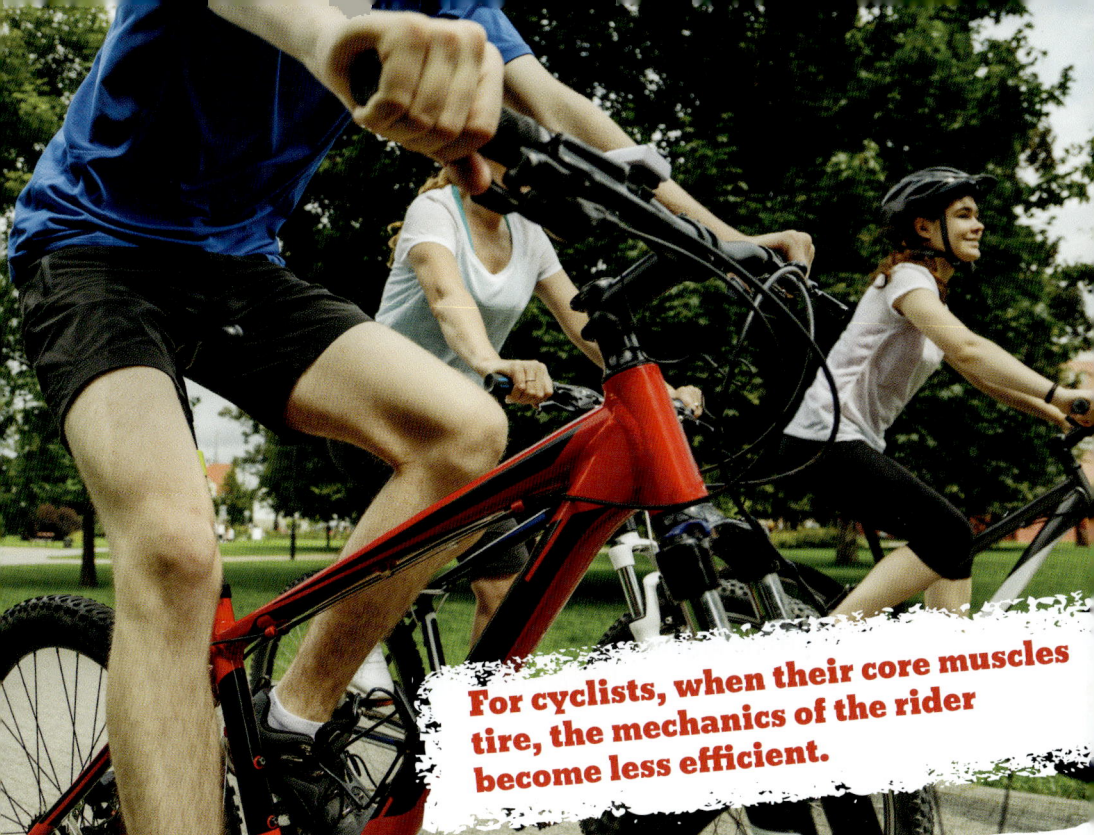

For cyclists, when their core muscles tire, the mechanics of the rider become less efficient.

Overall, the results suggest that direct, endurance-style core training has a limited effect on athletic performance, with its largest effect being injury prevention. Instead, you can improve core strength and stability through multi-joint weightlifting exercises such as Olympic lifts, squats, and deadlifts.

Injury Prevention

Developing a strong core can also prevent injury, as your entire body is connected along a kinetic chain. Studies show that poor core strength correlates with upper and lower extremity injuries. By asking our shoulders, hips, and neck muscles to do work they're not built for, they can get strained.

Research also shows that core stability exercises manage lower back pain. As you'll remember, the first job of core musculature is spinal stabilization. A weak core forces your lower back to take on loads, resulting in chronic low back pain. By developing core strength instead, you keep your spine in a safe position through movement.

When investigators examined the relationship between core stability and cycling output, they found that fatigued core muscles altered cycling mechanics. After a half-an-hour core workout, cyclists exhibited unnecessary ankle and knee motion. These results suggest that fatigue leads to compensatory movement patterns which over time could lead to overuse injury.

Improved Balance

The muscles of the core help to keep us upright on unstable surfaces. It all starts when we first learn to walk. Our bodies have to figure out how to transfer our weight from one leg to the next without falling over. During this process, our core muscles subtly contract and relax to correct for any errors. We are manipulating our body positioning to balance over the midfoot, battling gravity the entire time. By the time we're walking normally, our core receives this feedback and reacts without conscious thought.

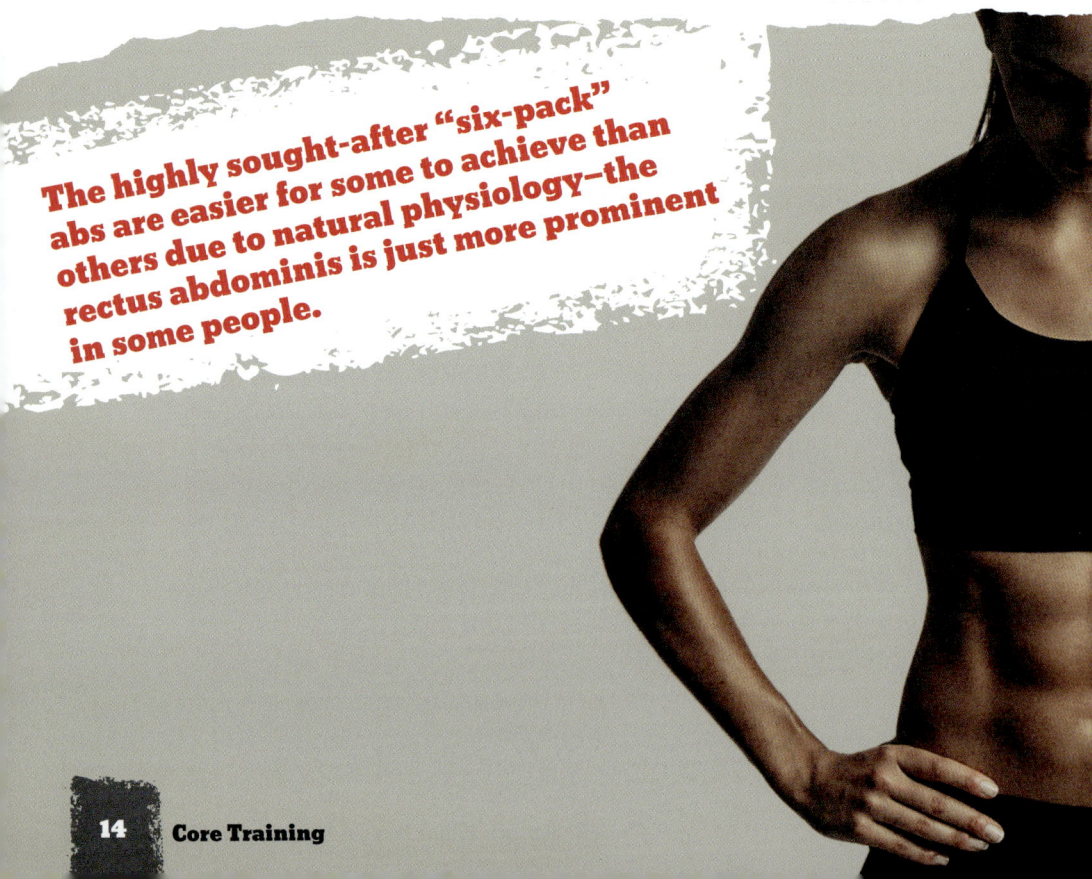

The highly sought-after "six-pack" abs are easier for some to achieve than others due to natural physiology—the rectus abdominis is just more prominent in some people.

This reflexive core activation has to be trained further every time new skills are acquired. Once walking is easy, we test how long we can balance on one leg. Then maybe you want to learn how to surf, changing the stability of the surface. Or maybe you're sprinting, cutting, and avoiding defenders—trying to maintain your position across multiple planes without getting tackled. If we can replicate these scenarios in the gym, we can train the patterns required for balance.

Physique Development

We can't ignore one of the most common reasons for training the core—to get visible abs. While all body types should be celebrated, lots of people want a six-pack. Core workouts help build the "mirror muscles" such as the rectus abdominis and obliques. However, a large part of muscle definition relies on diet. In addition, everybody is different. Some muscles naturally stick out more, while others take longer to reveal. Core training can certainly help you work toward a six-pack, but it's by no means the sole contributor. Diet, genetics, hormones, and other factors play a much larger role.

TEXT-DEPENDENT QUESTIONS

1. Name 2–3 global muscles of the core and describe how they contribute to athletic performance.

2. According to this chapter, which two muscle groups form the top and bottom of your core cylinder?

3. What role does the core play in balance as we're learning to walk?

RESEARCH PROJECT

Core training goes much further than looks, injury prevention, and athletic performance. In fact, it's one of the key elements in developing motor control as we grow into adults. Research core exercises for children (under age six) and put together a "workout plan" featuring 5–6 core exercises that are suitable for young kids.

WORDS TO UNDERSTAND

extension—an anatomical movement that increases the angle between two body parts

feed-forward reactions—actions within a controlled system that pass a signal from its source elsewhere in the environment without making adjustments for response

flexion—an anatomical movement that decreases the angle between two body parts

lateral flexion—flexion of the spine in a sideways manner

rotation—the movement of a body part around a single axis

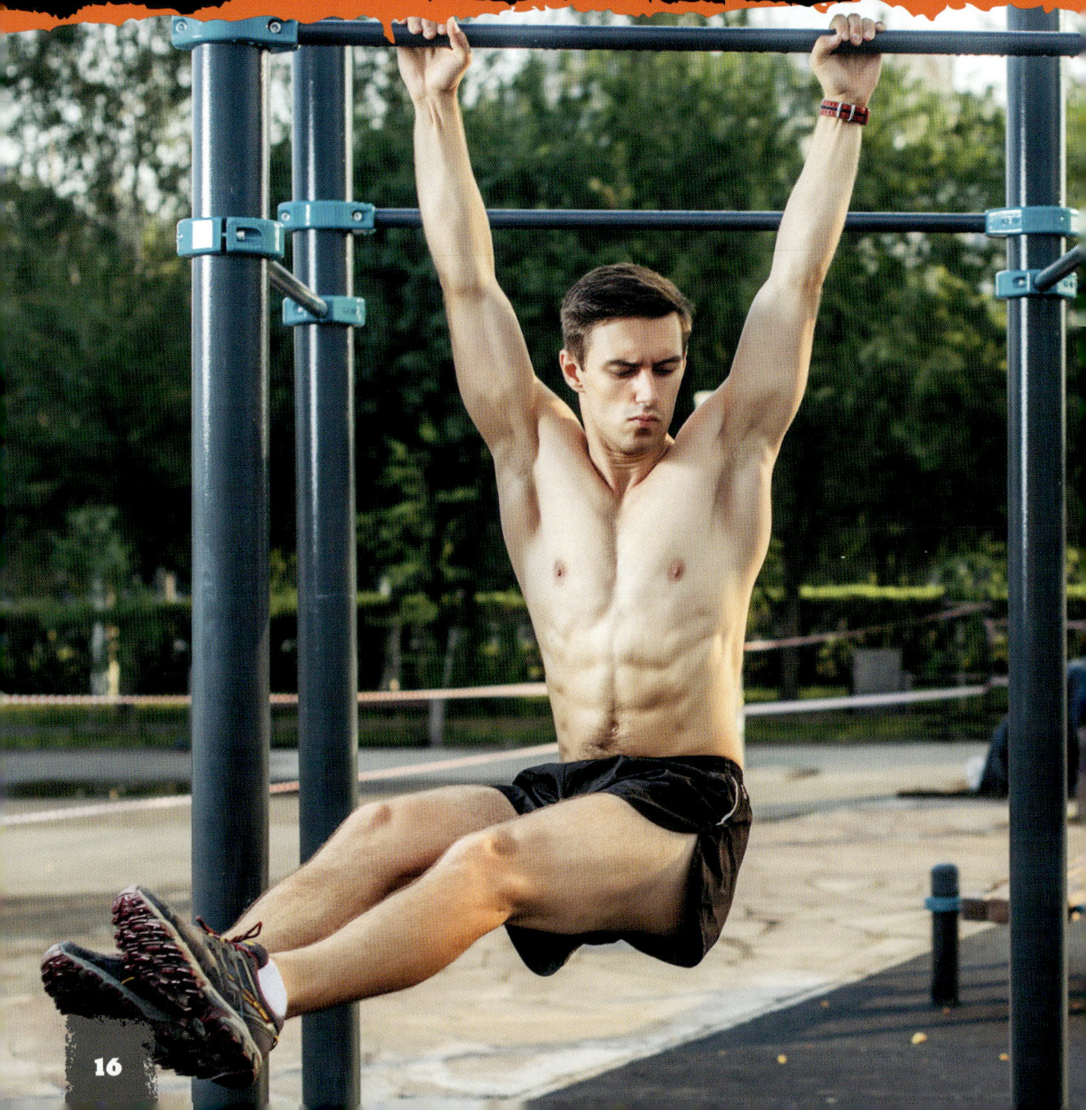

CHAPTER 2
CORE ANATOMY AND BIOMECHANICS

WHAT MUSCLES MAKE UP THE CORE?

Again, this is up for debate, but we're going to focus on the cylinder between your thorax and pelvis. Within your core, therefore, lie the following muscles as defined:

> Transverse abdominis (TVA)
> Multifidus
> Pelvic floor muscles
> Diaphragm
> Rectus abdominis
> External/internal obliques
> Iliopsoas
> Erector spinae
> Quadratus lumborum
> Glutes

Transverse Abdominis

TVA acts as a sort of corset around the midsection. Underneath the flashy roles of the rectus abdominis and obliques, the TVA lies deeper, directly compressing the ribs and pelvis for stability. It stems from the lateral inguinal ligament at the groin and the inner iliac crest, running up to the thoracolumbar fascia, and around through the middle of the abdomen.

Alongside the multifidi, the TVA controls postural **feed-forward reactions**. These reactions are often anticipatory in nature, as they

 Take a visual animated tour of the muscles of the inner core.

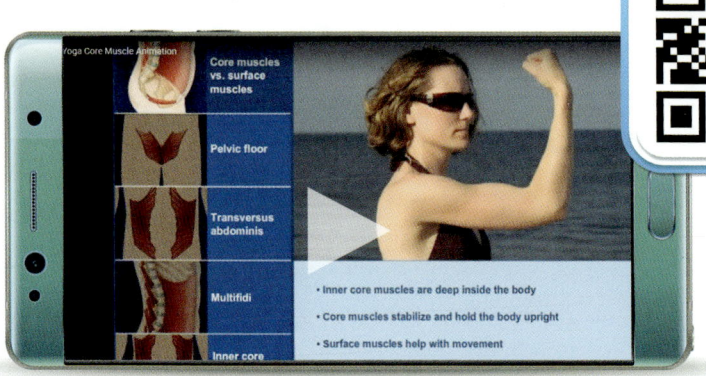

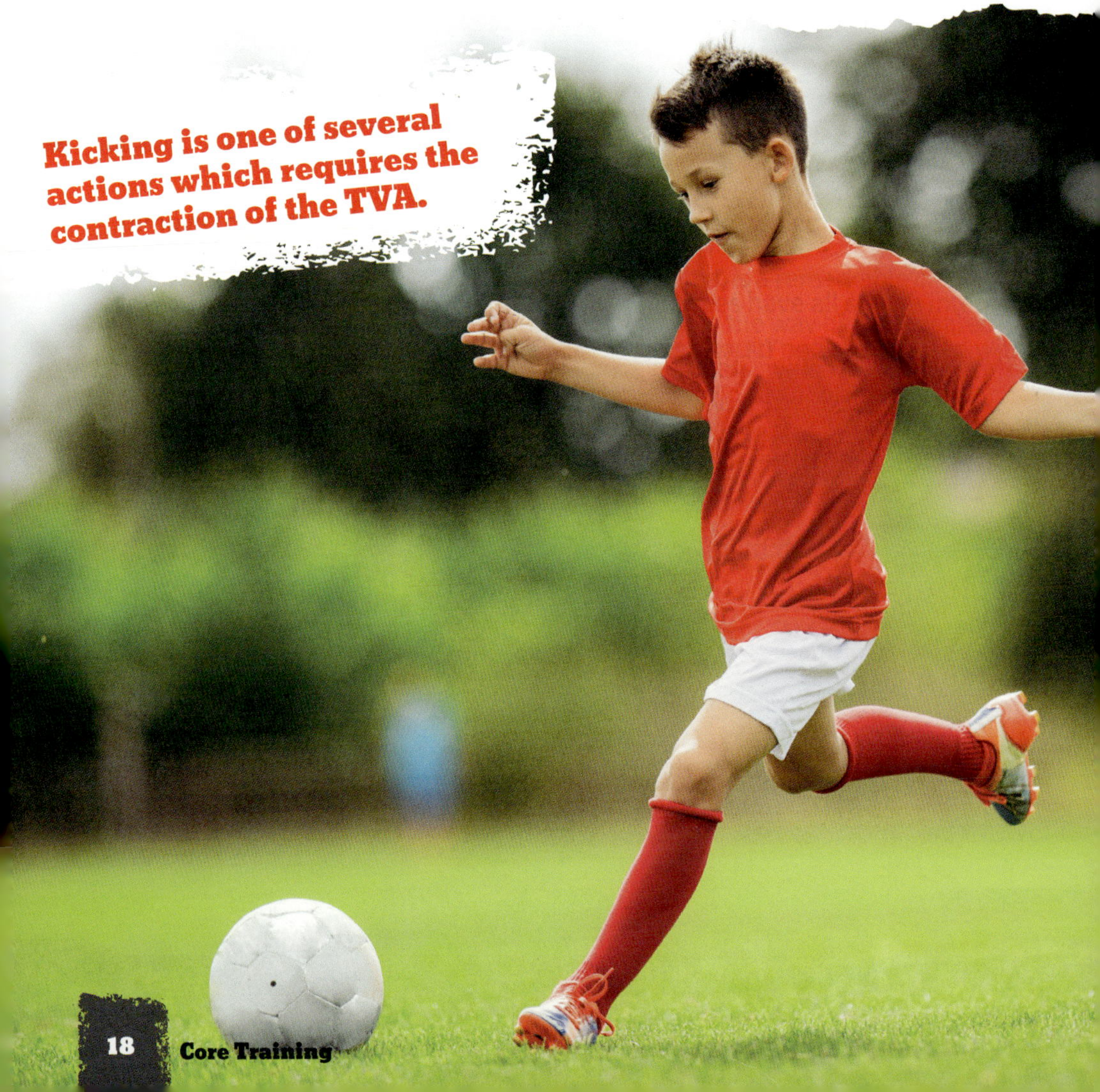

Kicking is one of several actions which requires the contraction of the TVA.

signal adjustments elsewhere in the environment without considering the response. Basically, your TVA contracts before movements such as throwing, kicking, or jumping to preemptively stabilize the spine. These contractions keep the pelvis and ribs aligned despite movement elsewhere, protecting the spinal cord from injury.

Multifidus

The multifidus acts as a sort of posterior version of the TVA. As a really deep muscle, it runs up and down the spine from the sacrum to the second cervical vertebrae, inserting at each vertebra along the way. As such, it helps stabilize each individual segment. While this might not seem life changing, no other muscles exert such specific control on the spinal segments. When other muscles pull against the spine to facilitate movement of the limbs, the multifidus acts as a counterbalance. Therefore, it keeps your spine safe through all sorts of activities, especially under load.

Pelvic Floor Muscles

Alongside the bottom of your pelvis lies a group of muscles that support the organs above. Your pelvic floor muscles control the bladder, bowels, and uterus (in women), but they also contribute to a stable core. Since they form the base of the cylinder, these muscles work in tandem with the multifidus and TVA to control spinal positioning during movement.

Diaphragm

On the other side of your core cylinder is your diaphragm. While we don't typically think of training this muscle, it's always working during exercise. Your diaphragm controls breathing, so you can't really ignore it. When you breathe in or contract your diaphragm, it moves downward, expanding your lungs with the help of your ribs. This diaphragmatic contraction creates a vacuum within the lungs, drawing air in for respiration. When it relaxes, its expansion pushes air out.

Although primarily under involuntary control, you can force your diaphragm to inhale or exhale. Try it now—take a deep breath, hold it, and blow it out as far as you can. That's controlling your diaphragm, and the importance of this will be apparent in the chapters that follow.

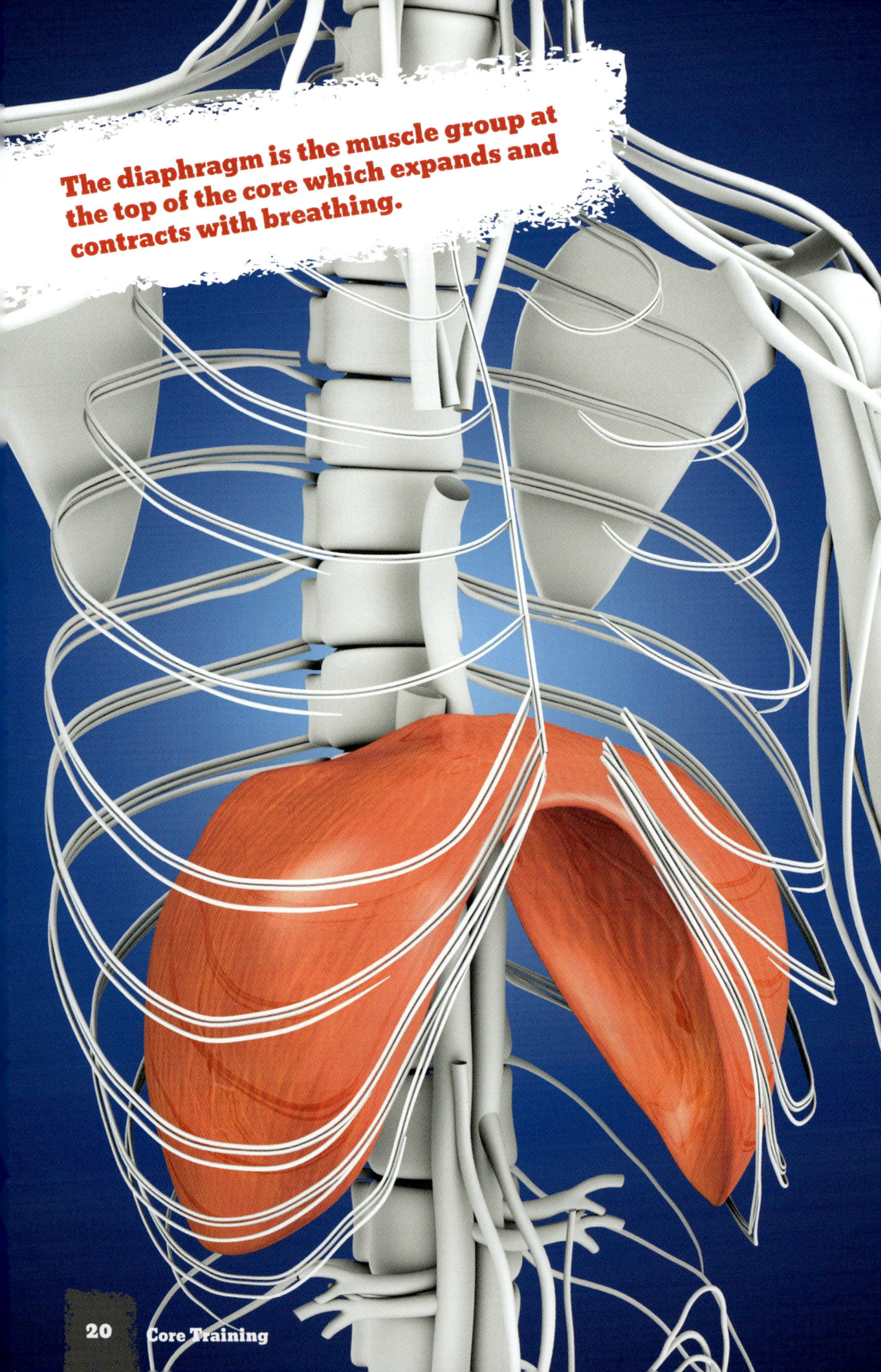

Rectus Abdominis

The rectus abdominis is the muscle people typically think of as abs. Its structure forms what's commonly called the six-pack, although there are technically 10 "packs"—five different pairs of parallel muscles. Running along the front of your midsection, the rectus abdominis originates at the pubic symphysis and inserts along the fifth through seventh ribs. In layman's terms, this means it covers the area from the hips to the sternum. The two sides of the abdominal wall are separated by the linea alba, forming the characteristic "packs," while other connective tissue divides them horizontally into distinct muscle bellies.

Besides just looking good, your rectus abdominis has a critical function. Its primary role is spinal **flexion**, but it also helps stabilize the trunk to combat movement. For example, doing a crunch works your rectus abdominis by tilting the ribs and the pelvis forward. In contrast, when one of those is locked in place, contraction of the rectus abdominis moves the other. Rectus abdominis activation becomes critical in keeping the ribs stacked over the pelvis for a neutral spine position.

External/Internal Obliques

The obliques assist with rotation and control your ability to separate your upper and lower halves. The internal oblique is located just on

THE FORGOTTEN COMPONENTS OF THE CORE—YOUR FASCIA

Surrounding your muscular tissue is a network of connective tissue known as fascia. Similar to the casing of a sausage, the fascia encloses and connects all muscles of the body. The thoracolumbar fascia, in particular, is a continuous membrane deep within your lower back. Due to its anatomy, it connects with the posterior ligaments of the lumbar spine. As such, it plays a supporting role in stabilizing the vertebrae and creating the necessary tension for safe movement.

the top of the TVA, running from the lumbar fascia, inguinal ligament, and the iliac crest up to the rib cage. Given its origin, insertion, and directionality of the fibers, contraction results in **rotation**. The internal obliques twist your body toward the same side—left internal obliques bring your midline to the left and vice versa on the right. They also assist with forced breathing, working in tandem with the diaphragm to expel air.

The external obliques, however, lie a bit more laterally. They originate around the 9th–12th ribs and insert onto the iliac crest, inguinal ligament, and pubic tubercle. This structure means the fibers run in the opposite direction to the internal obliques, while their contraction pulls the trunk in the opposite direction. Left-side external obliques rotate the body toward the right, and the right obliques pull toward the left. Opposing internal/external obliques, therefore, work in concert to help with dynamic rotation of the trunk. Both obliques also cause **lateral flexion** of the spine (think side bending) and assist the rectus abdominis with flexion.

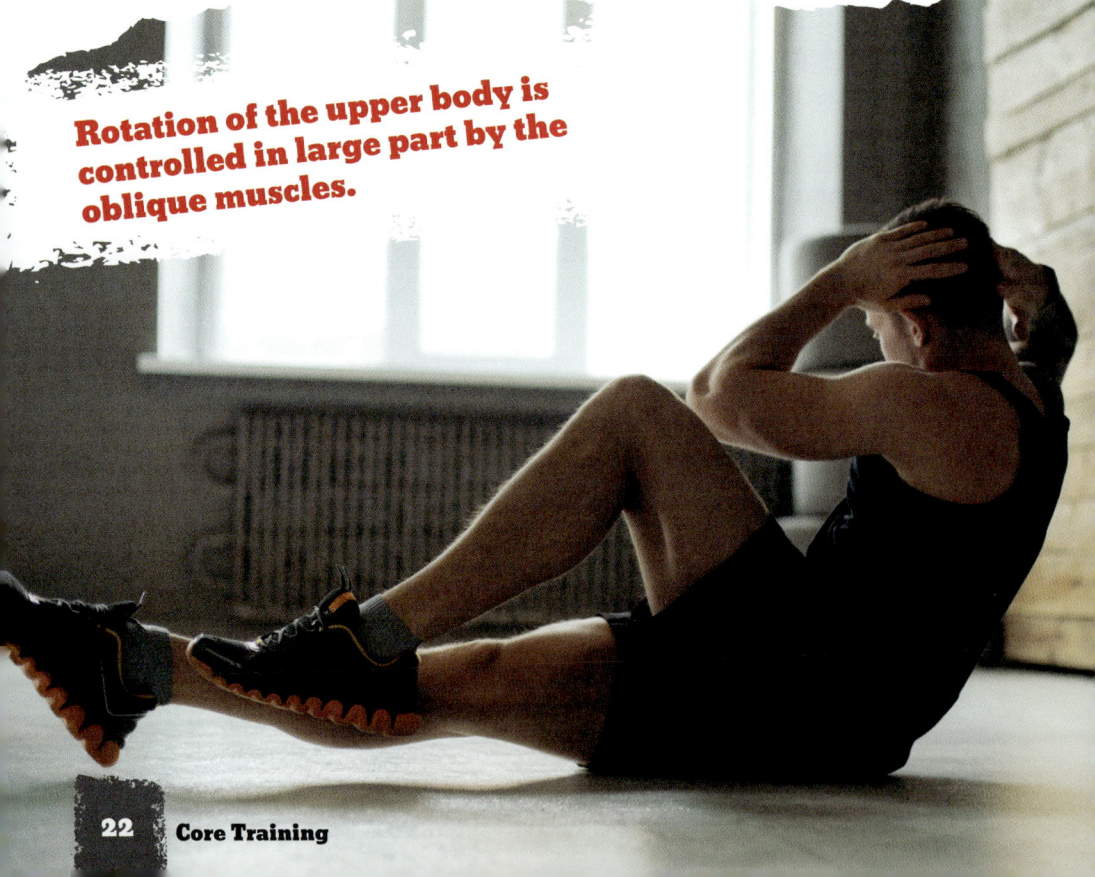

Rotation of the upper body is controlled in large part by the oblique muscles.

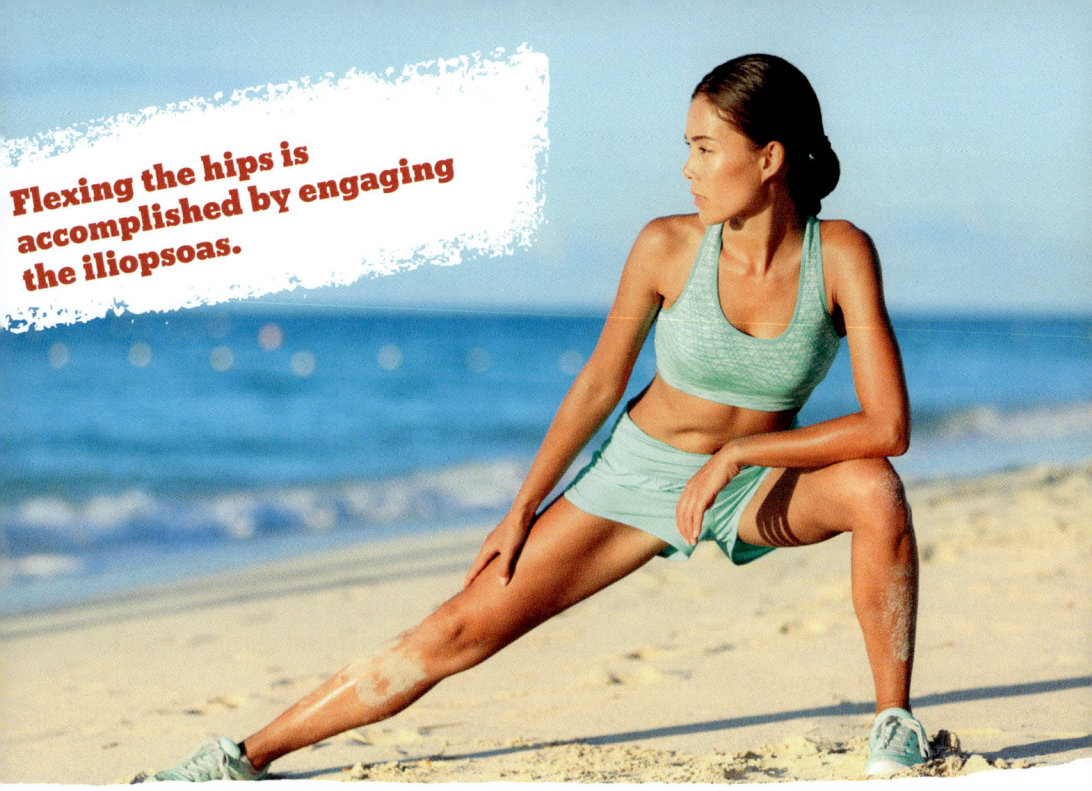

Flexing the hips is accomplished by engaging the iliopsoas.

Iliopsoas

The iliopsoas is a connection of two muscles: the iliacus and psoas major. Its primary function is to flex the hip, but it also flexes the trunk when the hips are fixed. As a postural muscle, it helps maintain normal spinal curvature. The psoas major originates at the T12–L4 vertebrae, merges with the iliacus, and inserts at the femur. The iliacus, on the other hand, originates from the superior iliac fossa, the iliac crest, and the sacrum. It runs along the inner side of your pelvic bones to attach to your upper leg. When combined, both muscles control lower extremity movement and play a huge role in pelvic tilt.

The iliopsoas tends to be one of the tighter muscles in the human body. That's because it's constantly contracted in a seated position. As we spend more and more of our lives sitting down, the iliopsoas gets negatively affected. Movement and balanced core training become critical to counterbalance any pelvic shift.

Erector Spinae

If you were to feel just along the sides of your spine, you'd be touching the erector spinae. Like two long ropes, these muscles travel up and down your back right next to the vertebral column. They're actually a group of three muscles and connective tissue—the iliocostalis, longissimus, and spinalis.

The first, the iliocostalis, runs from the top of your sacrum through fibrous tissue to three insertion points at the lumbar, thoracic, and cervical spine. The longissimus muscle is the largest of the three and runs slightly toward the middle of the back. Its fibers insert in the mid-back, cervical spine, and at the bottom of the skull. Finally, the spinalis is a shorter muscle originating higher up the spine and inserting at the thoracic and cervical spine as well as the base of the occipital bone in the skull.

Due to their extensive landscape across the back, it makes sense that these three muscles would maintain the curvature and posture of the spine. As a critical piece of the core, they not only stabilize the spine but also cause **extension** and lateral flexion of the back.

Quadratus Lumborum

Also called the QL, the quadratus lumborum muscles form the back of your abdominal wall. Originating on the side of your ilium (upper half of the pelvis), the QL runs up the back to attach between the bottom part of the 12th rib and the fourth lumbar vertebra (L4). Given that there's one on each side, contraction of one side causes lateral flexion of the spine or elevation of the pelvis. When both contract at the same time, the lower back extends.

Workouts rarely focus on the QL, but given its importance, this might be worth changing. As a counter to the iliopsoas, sitting regularly stretches out the QL while negating the need for stability. Accordingly, it is largely inactive. Even if you think about your posture while sitting, you'd constantly have to contract your QL to remain upright. Therefore, it's taking on either too much load or not enough load, putting you at a greater risk of lower back pain. We'll talk more about how regular core training can fix this issue in later chapters.

Glutes

The glutes consist of the gluteus maximus, minimus, and medius. Together, all three refer to large muscles stretching around the buttocks

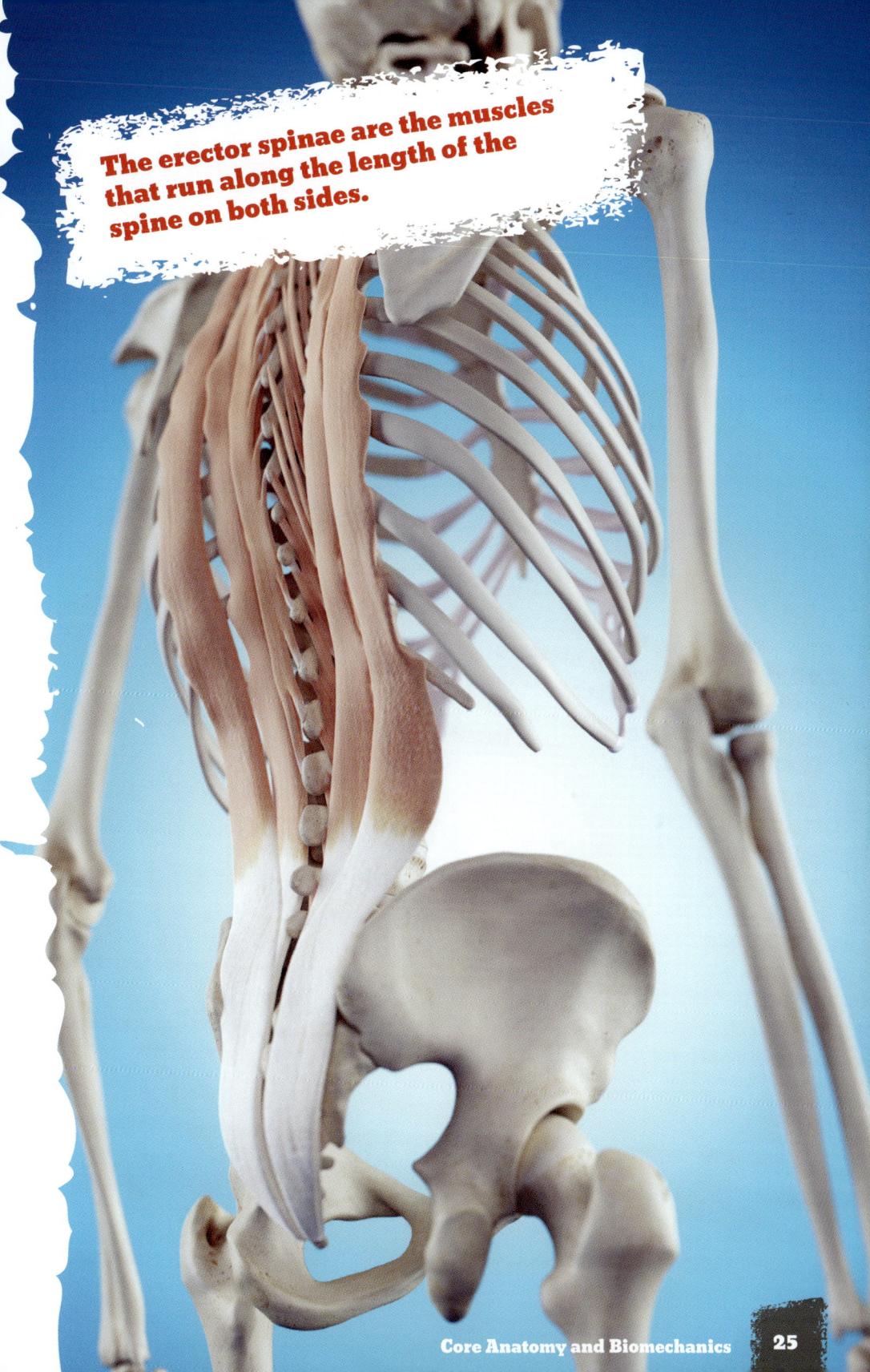

The erector spinae are the muscles that run along the length of the spine on both sides.

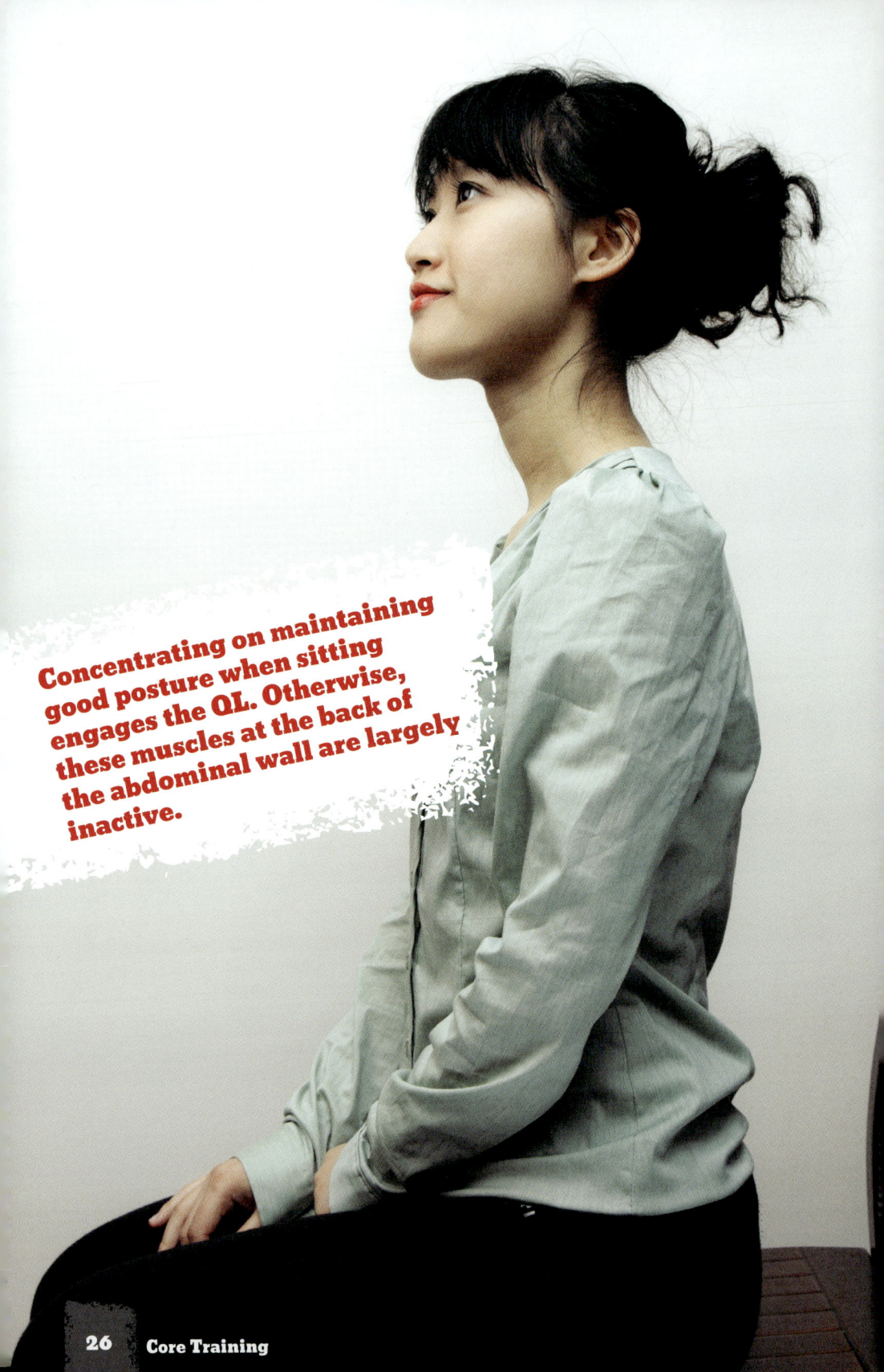

toward the femur. They work in concert to provide critical attachments for power and dynamic postural control.

The gluteus maximus, a large, thick muscle, lies just underneath the skin of your buttocks. It's the muscle most people try to train when they work their glutes. Originating at the iliac crest, sacrum, and coccyx, it inserts along your iliotibial band and upper femur. When activated, your gluteus maximus extends and externally rotates the hip.

The gluteus minimus, in contrast, hides just underneath the gluteus medius. It's a smaller counterpart to the gluteus maximus, starting at the ilium (pelvis) and attaching to your femur. It's a powerful assistant to the gluteus maximus in external rotation, especially when your glute max is busy with extension. Atop the gluteus minimus is your gluteus medius. This tiny muscle plays a huge role in dynamic stabilization of the lower body. When one leg is raised, both the gluteus medius and minimus act upon your femur to stabilize the leg.

TEXT-DEPENDENT QUESTIONS

1. Which four muscles make up the deep, inner core? Identify their primary roles.

2. What are spinal extension and flexion? Name two muscles responsible for each.

3. Which two muscles *primarily* contribute to the lower back pain caused by prolonged sitting?

RESEARCH PROJECT

As mentioned in the previous chapter, there's some debate on exactly which muscles make up the core. Given what you learned about the role of the core and anatomy/biomechanics of the muscles in this chapter, what other muscles could be considered part of the core? Research other muscles that attach to the trunk and come up with a solid argument as to why it should be included in core training.

Core Anatomy and Biomechanics

WORDS TO UNDERSTAND

dynamometer—an instrument that measures torque or rotational speed
isokinetic—referring to an action with a constant rate of speed, such as a muscle contraction
vestibular—refers to the sensory system of the inner ear responsible for balance and spatial awareness

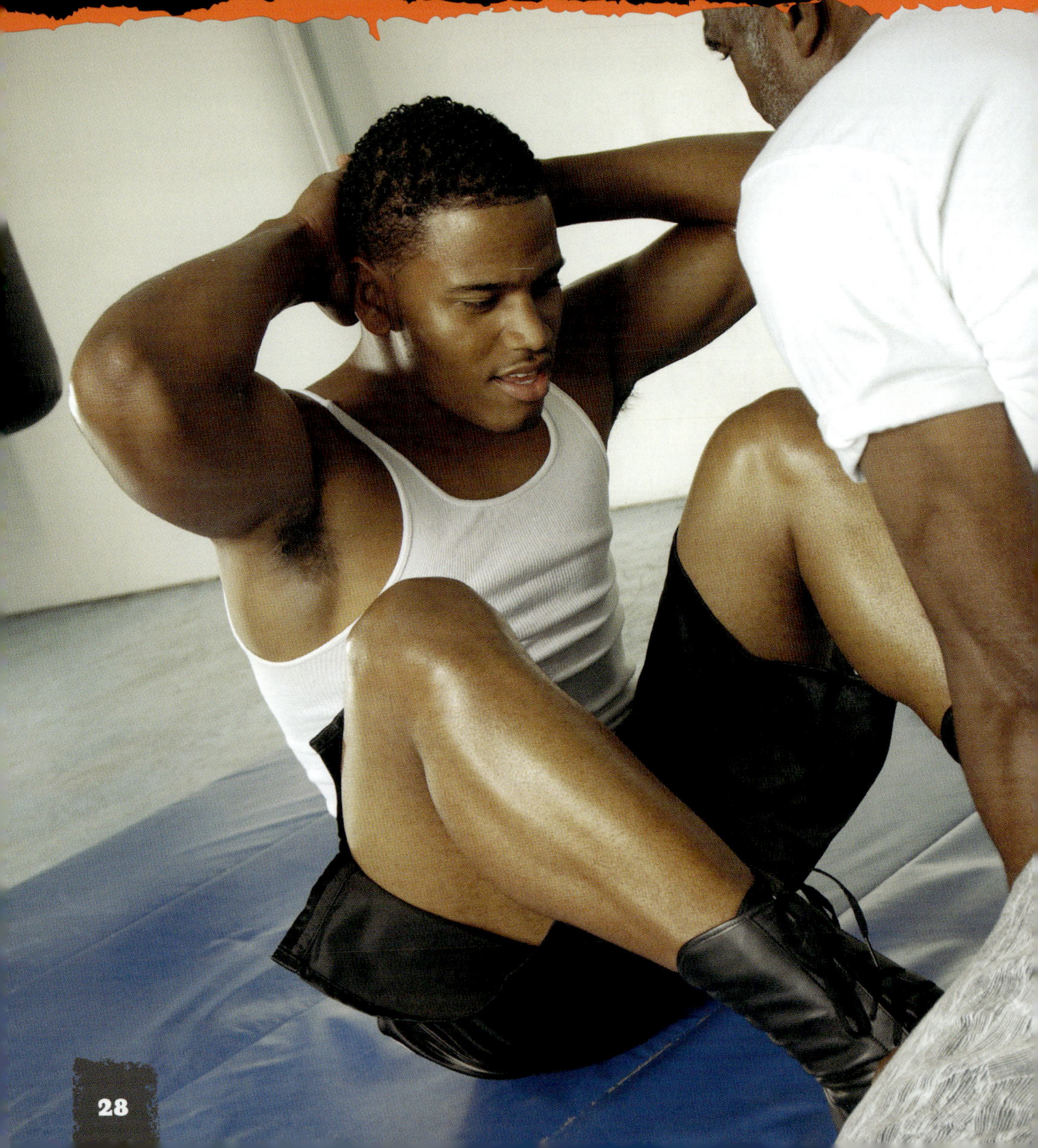

CHAPTER 3
ASSESSING THE CORE: STRENGTH VS. STABILITY

As discussed in earlier chapters, the core has two primary functions: stabilizing the spine and controlling movement. Unlike traditional lifts, however, you can't test core strength with a 1-rep max squat. So how do you measure the ability of your core musculature?

MEASURING CORE STRENGTH

Traditionally, core strength has been tested through a measure of endurance. For example, the military sit-up test requires a person to lie on his or her back, knees at 45° with feet flat on the floor. Testers count the maximum amount of times one can lift the torso from the floor to 90°. In fact, this only tests the endurance of the rectus abdominis and hip flexors, ignoring the rest of the core. However, since it's a standard, easy-to-implement testing protocol, the military, gym classes, and others regularly use this test to assess total core strength.

Static Assessments of Core Strength

Dr. Stuart McGill, one of the leading experts on spinal health and core training, expanded on the traditional sit-up test in 1995. Recognizing its limitations, he developed three alternative assessments of isometric core endurance across three planes of motion. As these three tests take a 360° view of core strength, many consider them a more beneficial assessment protocol.

 **Performing the trunk flexor test.**

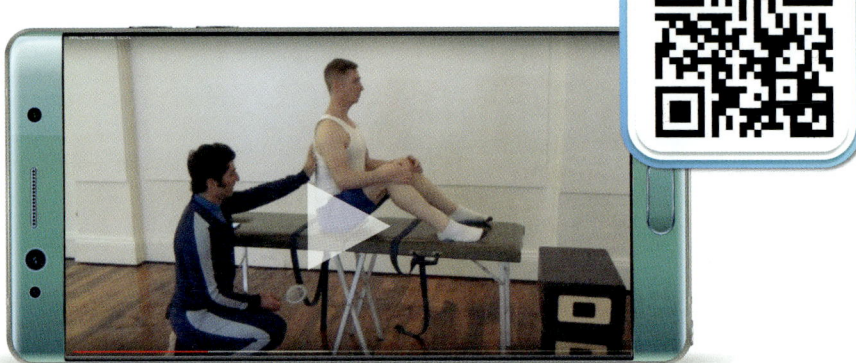

Trunk Flexor Test

The trunk flexor test (TFT) assesses the endurance of rectus abdominis by asking the participant to resist extension. To execute the TFT, sit on the floor with your knees and hips bent to 90°, arms folded across your chest. Grab a partner to stand behind you, holding something you can lean back against. Set up the supporting implement at a 60° angle to the floor, lean back against it, and then have your partner remove the support. Hold this leaned back position as long as possible, with the supporting implement now resting 10 inches away from your back. The test ends when you can no longer hold yourself up and your back reclines far enough to touch the support.

Trunk Extensor Test

The trunk extensor test (TET) primarily assesses the endurance of the erector spinae and multifidus. In order to execute the test, you'll need a partner and a bench to which you can secure your lower body. Locking the feet, knees, and hips in place, hang your torso off of the bench parallel to the floor. Your pelvic bones should sit just at the edge of the bench with arms crossed across your chest. Hold this position as long as possible until your partner sees you drop below horizontal.

Lateral Musculature Test (left and right)

Use the lateral musculature test to assess the endurance of your obliques, quadratus lumborum (QL), and transverse abdominis (TVA).

Performing the trunk extensor test.

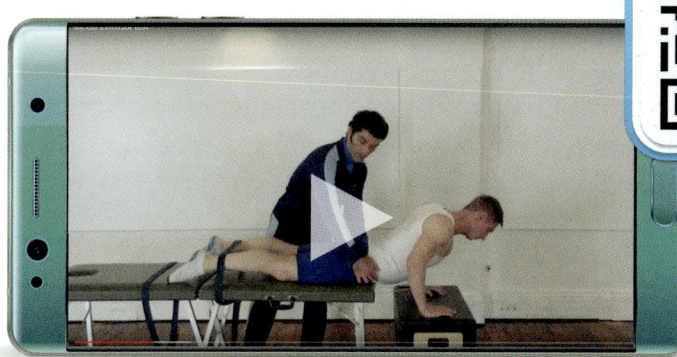

 Performing the lateral musculature test.

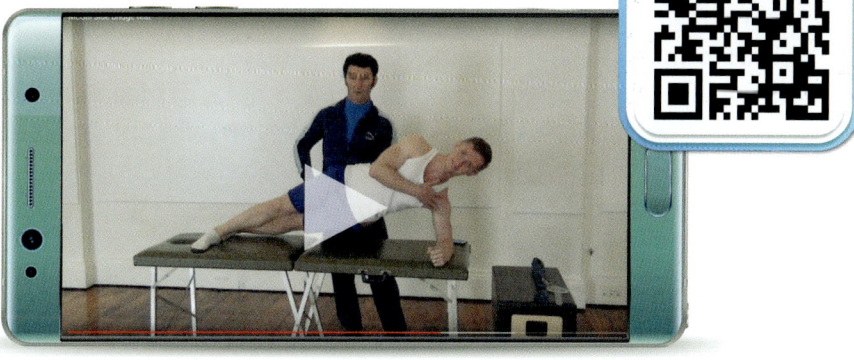

To execute the lateral musculature test, pick a side with which to lie on the floor. Keeping the legs extended, place the top foot slightly in front of your bottom foot for extra support. Lift the hips while supporting your weight on one elbow and the feet, creating a side bridge beneath your body. Keep your free arm across the chest and otherwise maintain a straight line between the head and the feet. Maintain this side bridge position as long as possible. The test ends when the body breaks from a straight line or the hips drop to the floor. Repeat on the other side.

Dynamic Assessments of Core Strength

One of the simplest ways to examine the core strength is standing postural alignment. Specifically, a trained eye will notice when the pelvis falls out of line with the lower extremities. As standing requires a small fight against gravity, balanced core engagement should equal a neutral pelvic tilt. However, if either anterior or posterior pelvic tilt occurs while standing, it could indicate weakness in the QL, TVA, obliques, or elsewhere.

Using Isokinetic Assessments of Strength

Isokinetic exercises require a constant rate of motion, meaning you can more accurately judge total muscular strength. As strength refers to force production, and force equates to mass times acceleration, keeping acceleration constant helps isolate the variable of strength. As such, isokinetic testing typically necessitates specialized equipment called **dynamometers**.

Isometric dynamometers set you up at a certain torso angle, predetermine the speed of movement, and record the force applied during the target range of motion. For example, to measure trunk flexion strength, align the machine's axis with the hip joint and bend forward with all your might. The same can be repeated with proper alignment through rotation, lateral flexion, and extension.

Medicine Ball Tests

Another common measure of core strength, especially in athletics, is the medicine ball toss. According to research carried out at the University of Pittsburgh, these tests don't show concurrent validity with isokinetic tests, highlighting once again the difficulty of defining core strength. However, strong test-retest reliability existed for each test, meaning that you can reliably repeat each test to measure changes in core strength.

Forward Medicine Ball Toss Test

The forward medicine ball toss assesses dynamic trunk flexion, that is, how much power your rectus abdominis and hip flexors can produce. To perform the test, complete the following steps:

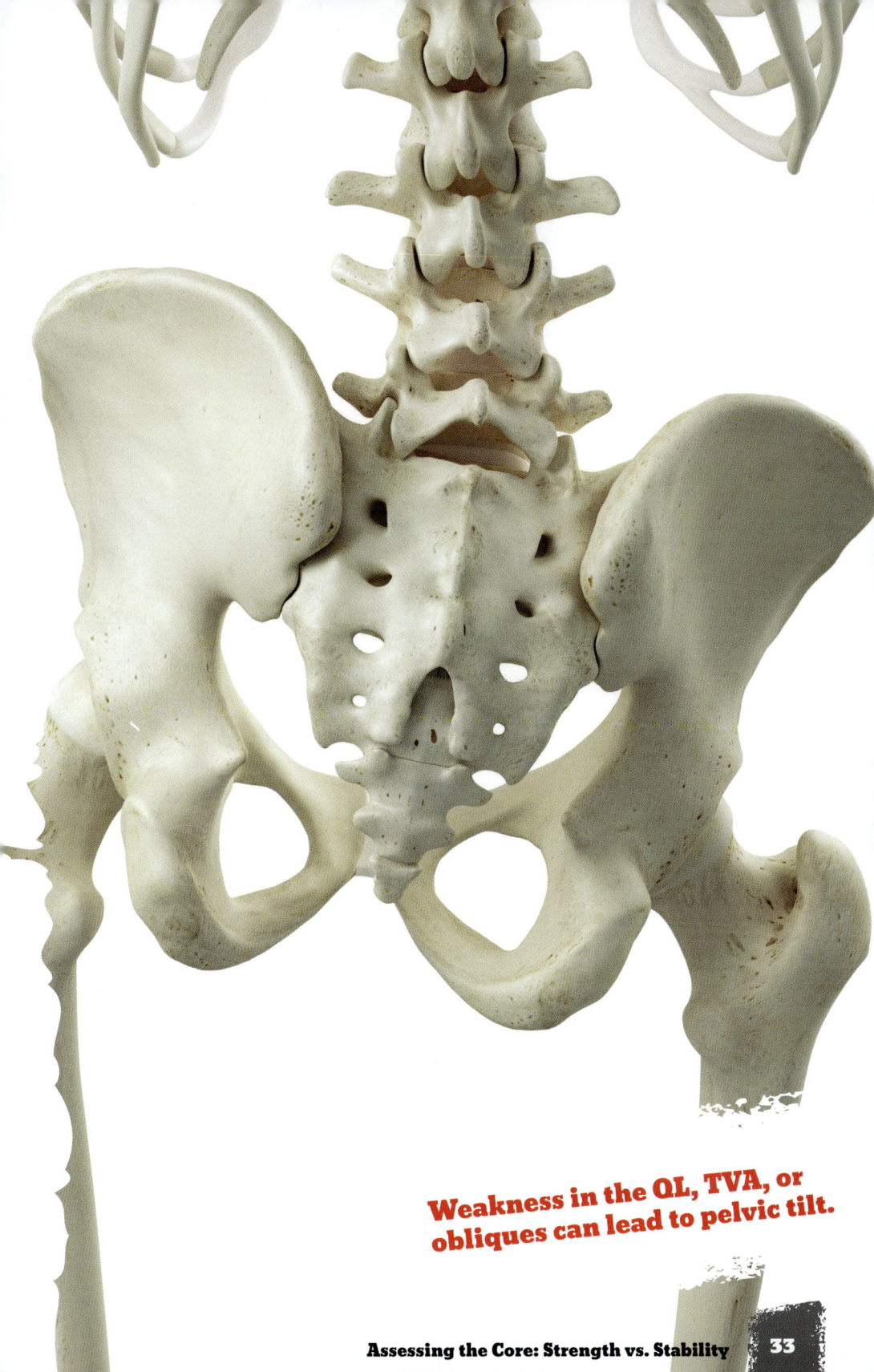

Weakness in the QL, TVA, or obliques can lead to pelvic tilt.

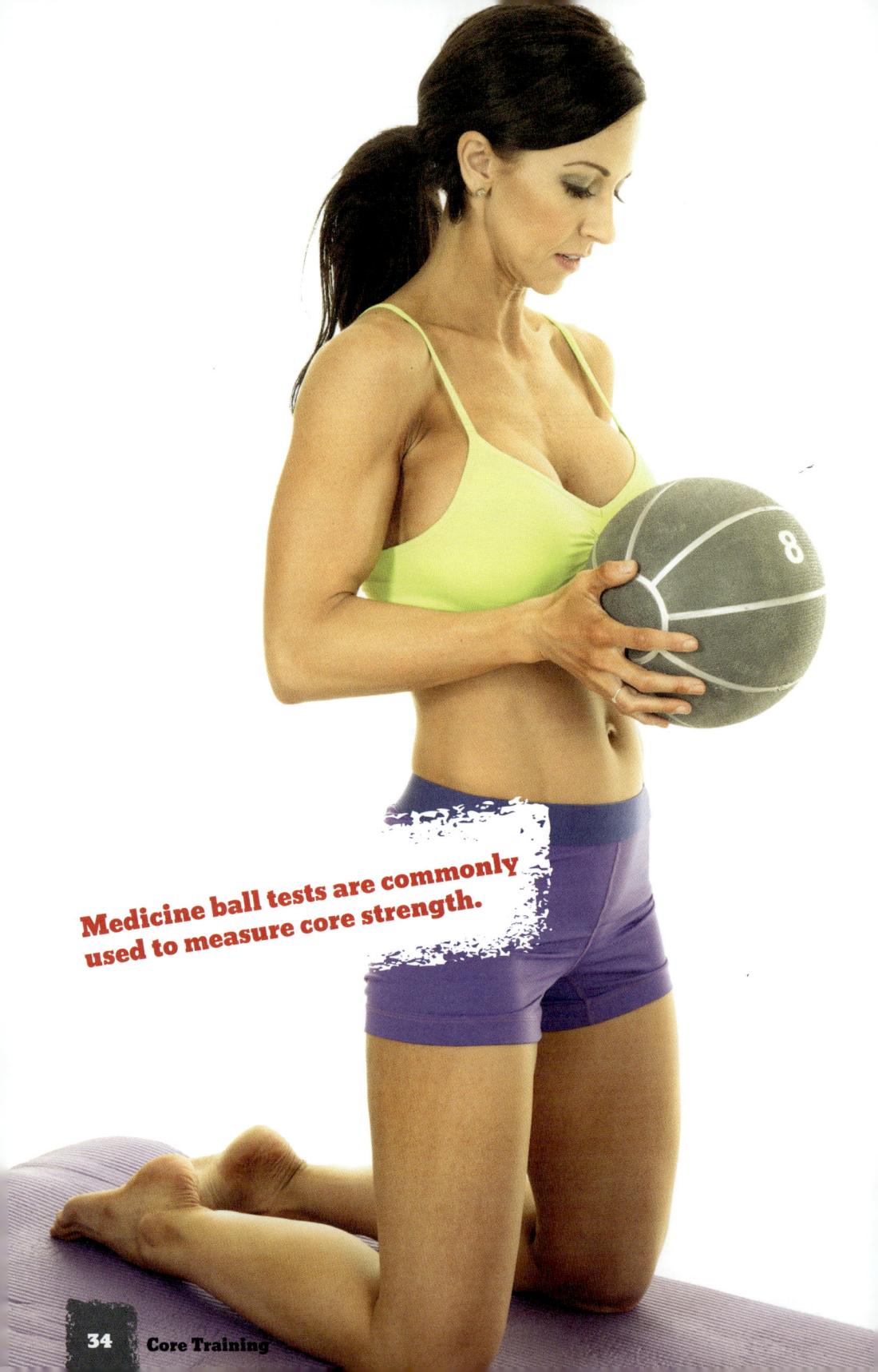

Medicine ball tests are commonly used to measure core strength.

1. Kneel in a tall position atop a mat on the floor, keeping the knee angle at 90°. Keep your hips and spine stacked directly atop each other. Make sure to place a piece of tape or other marker at the edge of your knees.
2. Raise a medicine ball overhead with both hands, palms facing inward, locking the elbows in extension to avoid triceps interference.
3. To begin the throw, extend the hips as far as comfort will allow while staying tall. Flex the hips and spine to fold forward, and release the ball at the top. The aim is to generate enough force through the abdominals to throw the ball as far as possible.
4. Measure the distance from the knees to the point at which the medicine ball makes initial contact with the floor and compare across future tests.

Backward Medicine Ball Toss Test

The backward medicine ball toss test measures the dynamic strength of the trunk extensors. Specifically, it looks at power output from the erector spinae, glutes, QL, and multifidus. To execute the test, follow these steps:

1. Kneel in a tall position atop a mat on the floor, keeping the knee angle at 90°. Keep your hips and spine stacked directly atop each other. Make sure to place a piece of tape or other marker at the edge of your knees.
2. Raise a medicine ball overhead with both hands, palms facing inward, locking the elbows in extension to avoid triceps interference.
3. To begin the throw, flex the hips and lumbar spine as far forward as comfortable. The hips can drop to touch the calves so you're fully bent over. Make sure to keep arms locked out overhead.
4. Then, rapidly extend the hips and spine, releasing the ball behind you at the top. The goal should be to throw the medicine ball as far as possible.
5. Measure the distance from the knees to the point at which the medicine ball makes initial contact with the floor and compare across future tests.

Rotational Medicine Ball Toss Test

The rotational medicine ball toss test is an assessment of rotational power, that is, the strength of your obliques. Similar to the other medicine ball toss tests, you'll start by kneeling on the floor. However, instead of throwing forward or backward, you're tossing the ball laterally. To execute this test, follow these steps:

1. Kneel in a tall position atop a mat on the floor, keeping the knee angle at 90°. Keep your hips and spine stacked directly atop each other. Make sure to place a piece of tape or other marker at the edge of your knees.
2. Position the shoulders in neutral with no flexion or extension, resting just by your side. Bend the elbows to 90° to hold the medicine ball with both hands in front of you, keeping the arms locked at your side.
3. To begin the throw, rotate as far as you can to one side, away from the direction you'll be throwing. For example, if you're throwing to the right, rotate as far as possible to the left. Make sure to maintain that arm position to isolate the trunk.
4. Rapidly rotate back to center. As the spine returns to neutral, release the ball and throw it as far as possible. Measure the distance traveled between the starting tape and the medicine ball's initial point of contact with the floor. Repeat on the other side and retest as necessary to assess changes in strength.

MEASURING CORE STABILITY

While any of the static assessments of core strength could be used to test stability, total core stability emerges during unilateral exercises. One of the best measures of core stability, therefore, is the unilateral hip bridge endurance test. The hip bridge commonly measures lumbar stabilization, and when performed unilaterally, it requires significant neuromuscular control. In one exercise, you can test anti-flexion, anti-extension, and anti-rotation.

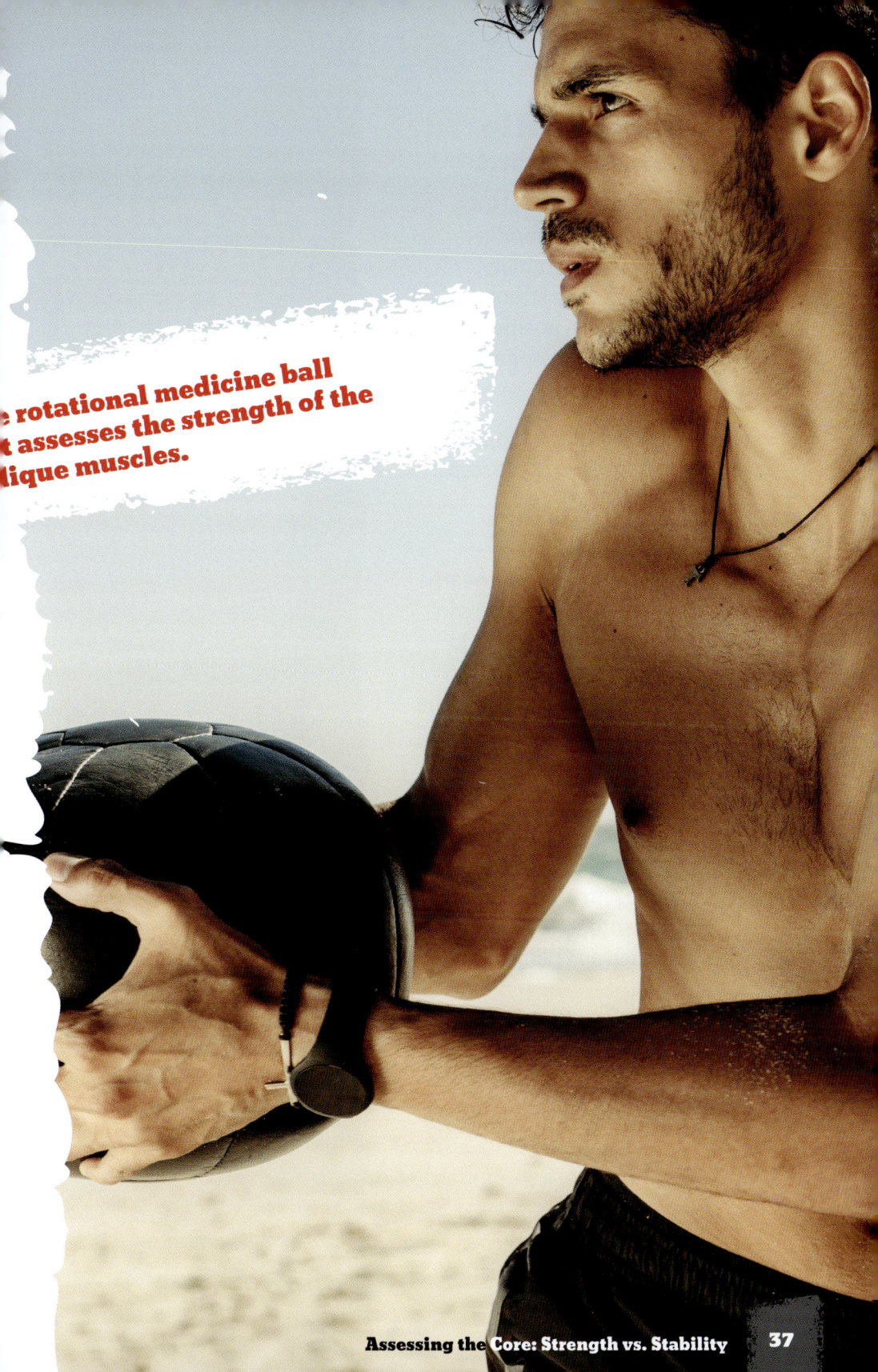

The rotational medicine ball test assesses the strength of the oblique muscles.

The Unilateral Hip Bridge Assessment

To begin this test it's critical to start with a bilateral hip bridge. People who lack core stability, motor control, or glute strength will struggle with this position. If this is the case, do not progress to unilateral assessments.

To execute the unilateral hip bridge endurance test, follow these steps:

1. Lie flat on the floor with a neutral spine with the knees bent and heels just underneath the hips. Keeping your heels in contact with the floor, extend the hips by squeezing the glutes. Make sure not to arch the lower back, overextending the lumbar spine.

2. Once you've executed a bilateral hip bridge, keep one foot on the floor while extending one leg straight out. Aim to keep thighs next to each other, keeping both hips extended and parallel with the ground.

3. Maintain this position as long as possible. The test ends when hips start to drop past 0° of extension or one side rotates toward the floor.

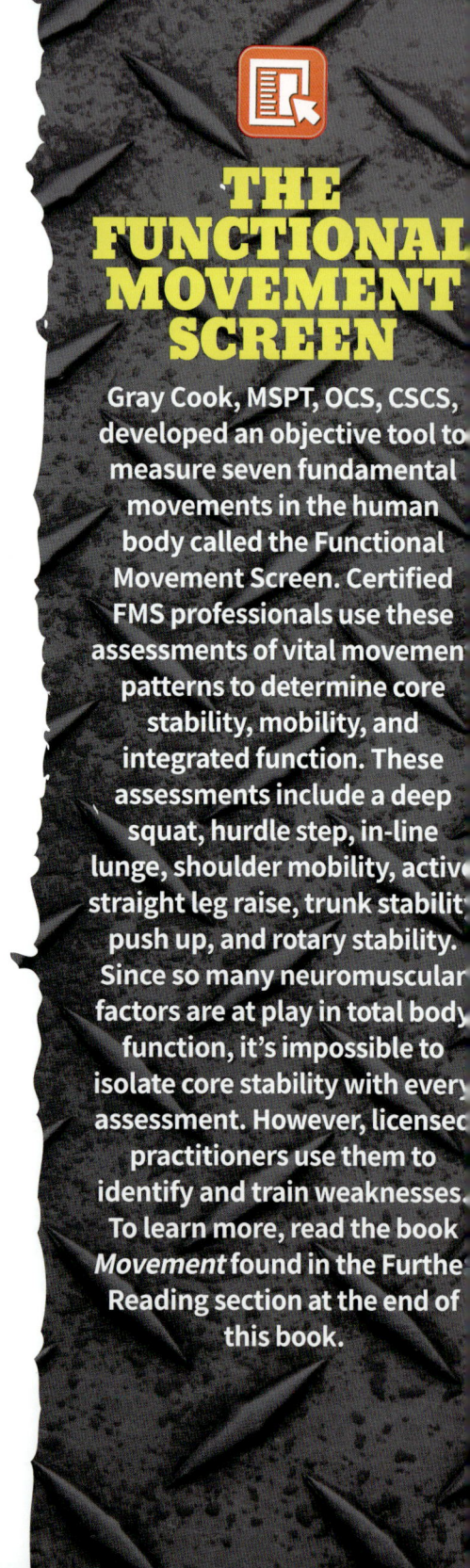

THE FUNCTIONAL MOVEMENT SCREEN

Gray Cook, MSPT, OCS, CSCS, developed an objective tool to measure seven fundamental movements in the human body called the Functional Movement Screen. Certified FMS professionals use these assessments of vital movement patterns to determine core stability, mobility, and integrated function. These assessments include a deep squat, hurdle step, in-line lunge, shoulder mobility, active straight leg raise, trunk stability push up, and rotary stability. Since so many neuromuscular factors are at play in total body function, it's impossible to isolate core stability with every assessment. However, licensed practitioners use them to identify and train weaknesses. To learn more, read the book *Movement* found in the Further Reading section at the end of this book.

The Single-Leg Balance/Squat Test

The single-leg balance/squat assessment takes a more global look at dynamic core stability. It measures the core's ability to balance weight over a base of support during movement. As it involves all muscles of the hip, however, there are lots of factors at play. Ankle mobility, lower leg strength, **vestibular** issues, or anatomical restrictions will affect results. Still, the single-leg squat provides an overall look at one's ability to apply stability in real-life situations.

To execute the single-leg balance test, begin by standing tall with hands on the hips. Slowly lift one leg a few inches off of the ground. Keep a

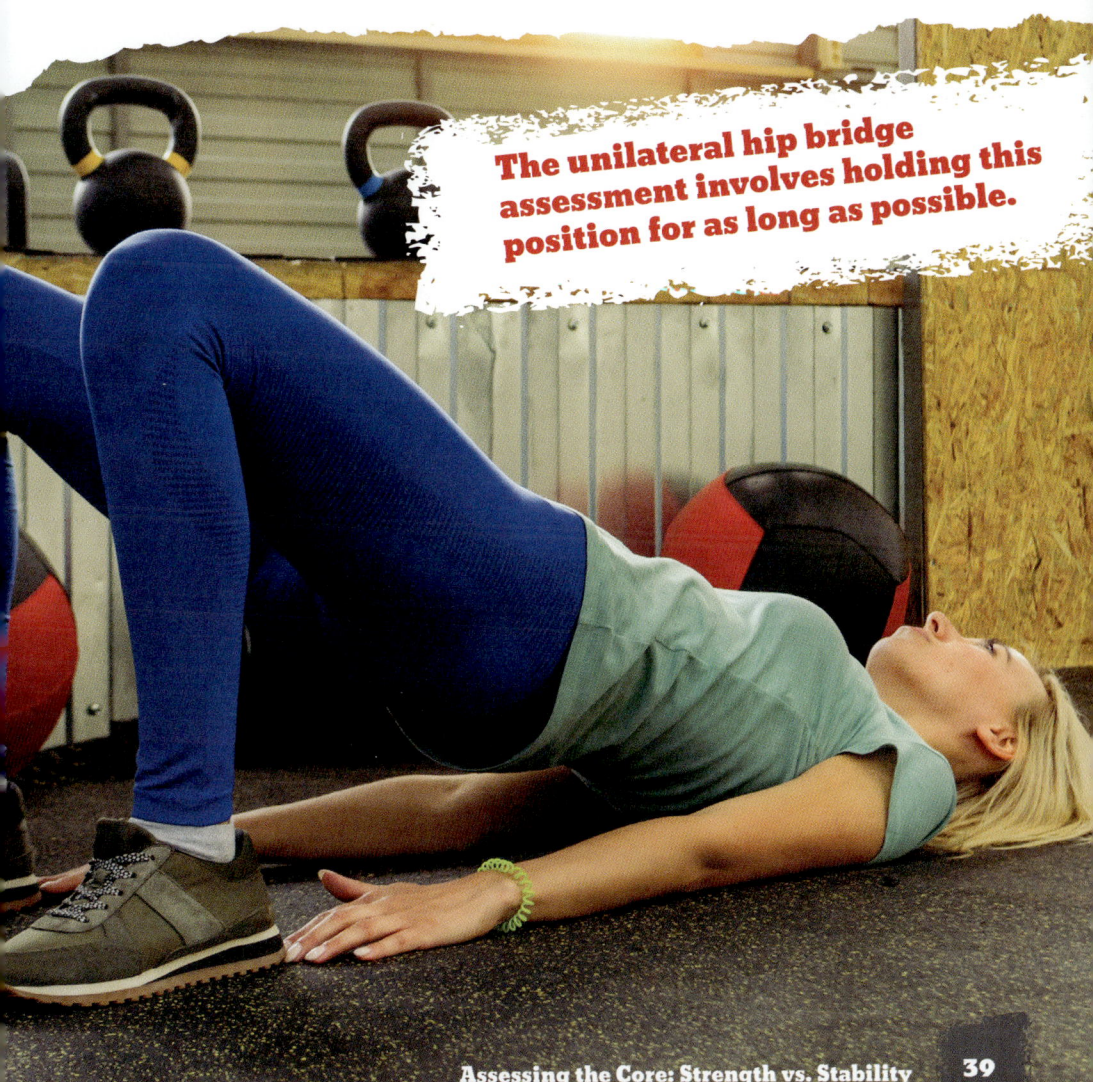

The unilateral hip bridge assessment involves holding this position for as long as possible.

> **The squat position is the progression of the single-leg balance assessment test.**

slight bend in the knee and balance your weight over the midfoot of the standing leg. Maintain this position without falling, removing your hands or placing the other foot on the ground for as long as possible.

To progress this test, you could close one or both eyes. To make it more dynamic, add a squat element. Watch for any instability as you lower into a single-leg squat position and stand up. However, all of these tests are advanced assessments of stability and should only be performed if other measures are too easy.

TEXT-DEPENDENT QUESTIONS

1. Based on the assessments discussed in this chapter, which core stability test would you recommend for a complete beginner?
2. What's the issue with using only the maximum sit-up assessment for core strength?
3. What are the primary limiting factors when assessing core strength?

RESEARCH PROJECT

Choose one of the "Big 3" exercises—the squat, the deadlift, or the bench press—and identify the role the core plays in their execution. Which muscles of the core are used? Which core assessment do you think would correlate with performance in the lift? Why? Write a 500-word essay on assessing core strength for that lift, indicating which test you would use and how you would measure improvements.

WORDS TO UNDERSTAND

afferent neurons—neurons that carry sensory information from the body to the central nervous system (CNS)

anticipatory postural adjustments—core musculature activations that precede voluntary movement

efferent neurons—neurons that carry signals from the CNS to muscles and other organs within the body

prone—a position lying flat and face downward

supine—a position lying on one's back and facing upward

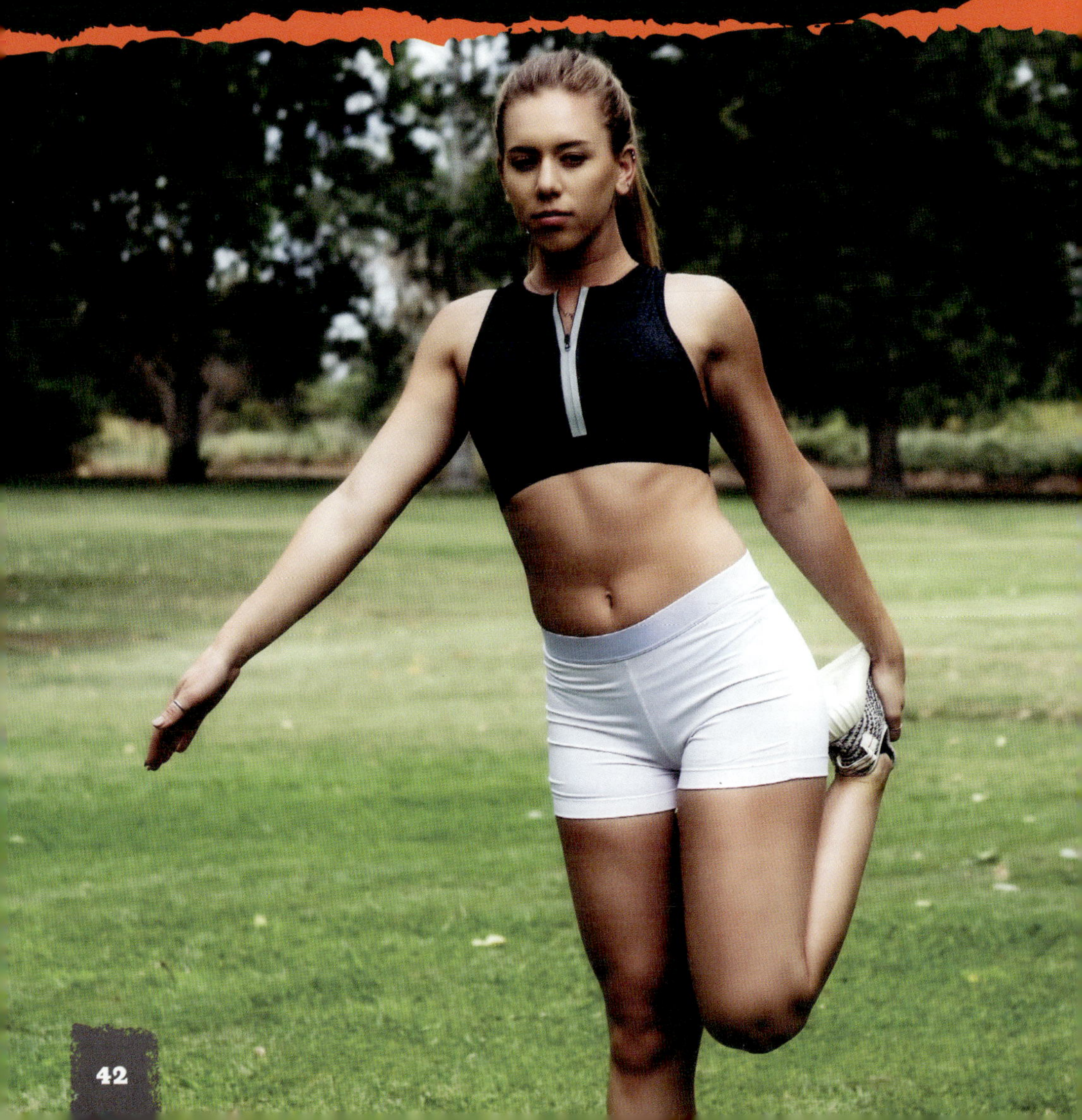

CHAPTER 4
THE SCIENCE OF CORE STABILITY

In order to understand the science of core stability, we have to establish an initial position. It's hard to call something "stable" if you don't know what the original posture is supposed to look like. Theoretically, the more intra-abdominal pressure you can create, the more stability you can achieve. However, Hodges and Cholewicki give us the definition: "the ability to maintain the desired trajectory despite kinetic, kinematic, or control disturbances."

CREATING A STABLE BASE THROUGH JOINT CENTRATION

Gray Cook, the founder of Functional Movement Systems, a world-renowned movement-screening company, considers the core to have four positions of neurodevelopment. Basically, the human body has to cope with variations of being **supine, prone**, kneeling, and standing. In each position, each joint has its ideal angle to manage maximal load with minimal strain. This also applies to variations. For example, a squat, as a variation of standing, comes with ideal joint positioning to absorb and recreate force. Core stability, therefore, can be defined as the reflexive neuromuscular activity to maintain and transition between these ideal positions.

Every single human has slightly different anatomy. So what's ideal for you might not be ideal for your best friend, which might not be ideal for your favorite athlete. However, a consensus exists around restricting excessive spinal movement during limb activity. With so much going on in the human body, this is surprisingly difficult to do. So difficult, in fact, that simply breathing incorrectly can throw us off.

THE ROLE OF DIAPHRAGMATIC BREATHING

Breathing in and out requires diaphragmatic contraction and relaxation. The human body is built for this, as the midsection opens up just beneath the rib cage to allow for the natural rise and fall of the breath. Interestingly enough, it's become a lost art. More often than not, individuals rely on the expansion of their chest to breathe. While this certainly won't kill you, it does alter the position of the rib cage, which is attached to the spine, to which all muscles of the core attach. Since everything is so interconnected, flaring the ribs shifts us out of an ideal position. Diaphragmatic breathing, therefore, can be considered the foundation of core stability.

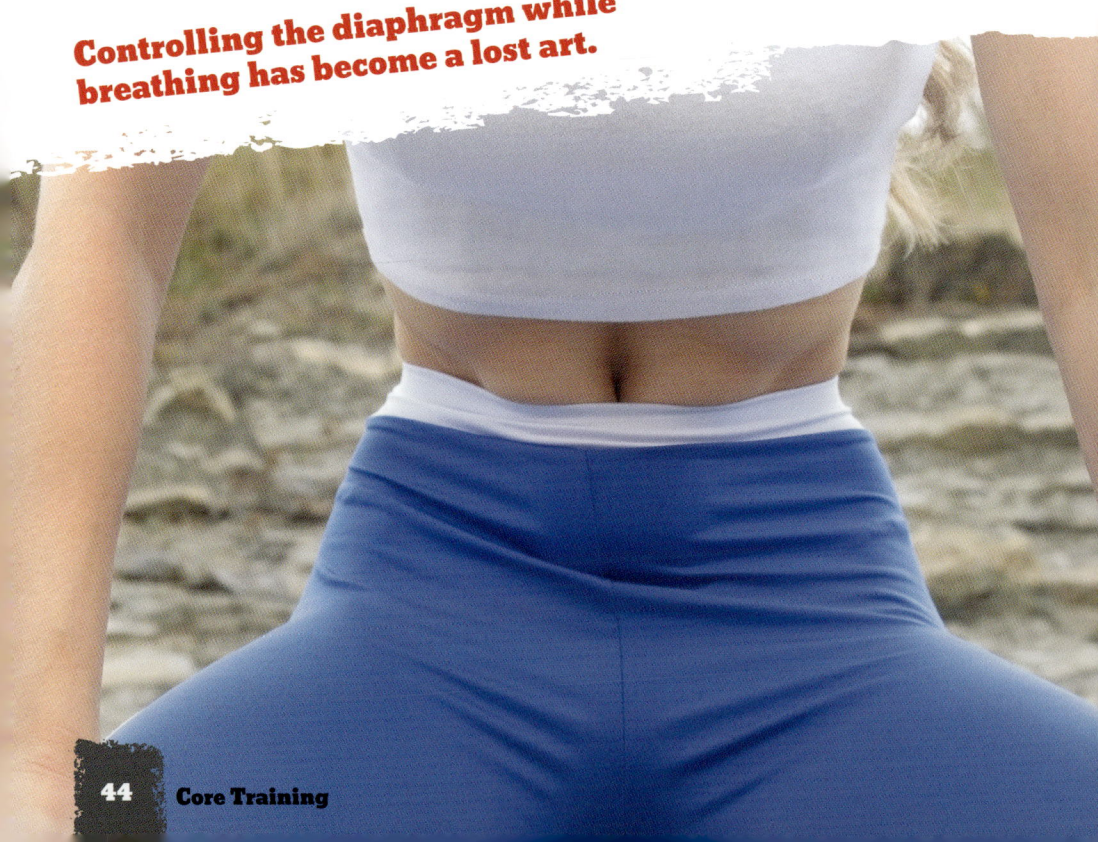

Controlling the diaphragm while breathing has become a lost art.

However, it should be noted that when transitioning to higher developmental positions—that is, supine to prone and definitely supine to standing—diaphragmatic breathing becomes more difficult. This is because we're increasingly reliant on our core musculature to keep us upright. Rapid postural changes cause the diaphragm to contract in an effort to control postural stability. In a sense, your subconscious neuromuscular control is busy doing other things. Therefore, it's important to train diaphragmatic breathing through increasingly higher core activation.

THE CORE'S ROLE IN STABILIZING AGAINST MOVEMENT

According to the research by M. M. Panjabi, Professor Emeritus of Orthopaedic Medicine at Yale University, core stabilization includes three interdependent systems. Those systems include passive, active, and neural control. While we don't often train the passive system, it refers to static tissue such as vertebrae, spinal disks, and the ligaments that attach muscles to joints. Core training is based on the integrity of these tissues. If the foundation is off, it completely alters core function. Therefore, a professional should always assess any pain or mobility issues to reassure that there aren't any structural abnormalities.

The active system of the core features muscles that dynamically stabilize the spine and your extremities. These muscles also transmit information across the torso about movement further down or up the kinetic chain. The core, therefore, plays a pivotal role in transferring power from the ground to the upper extremities.

The incoming and outgoing signals relayed to the nervous system ultimately maintain core stability. No muscles, neither passive nor active nervous interactions, act independently. At the end of the day, the entire core engages in response to specific movements to protect the spine and optimize the power.

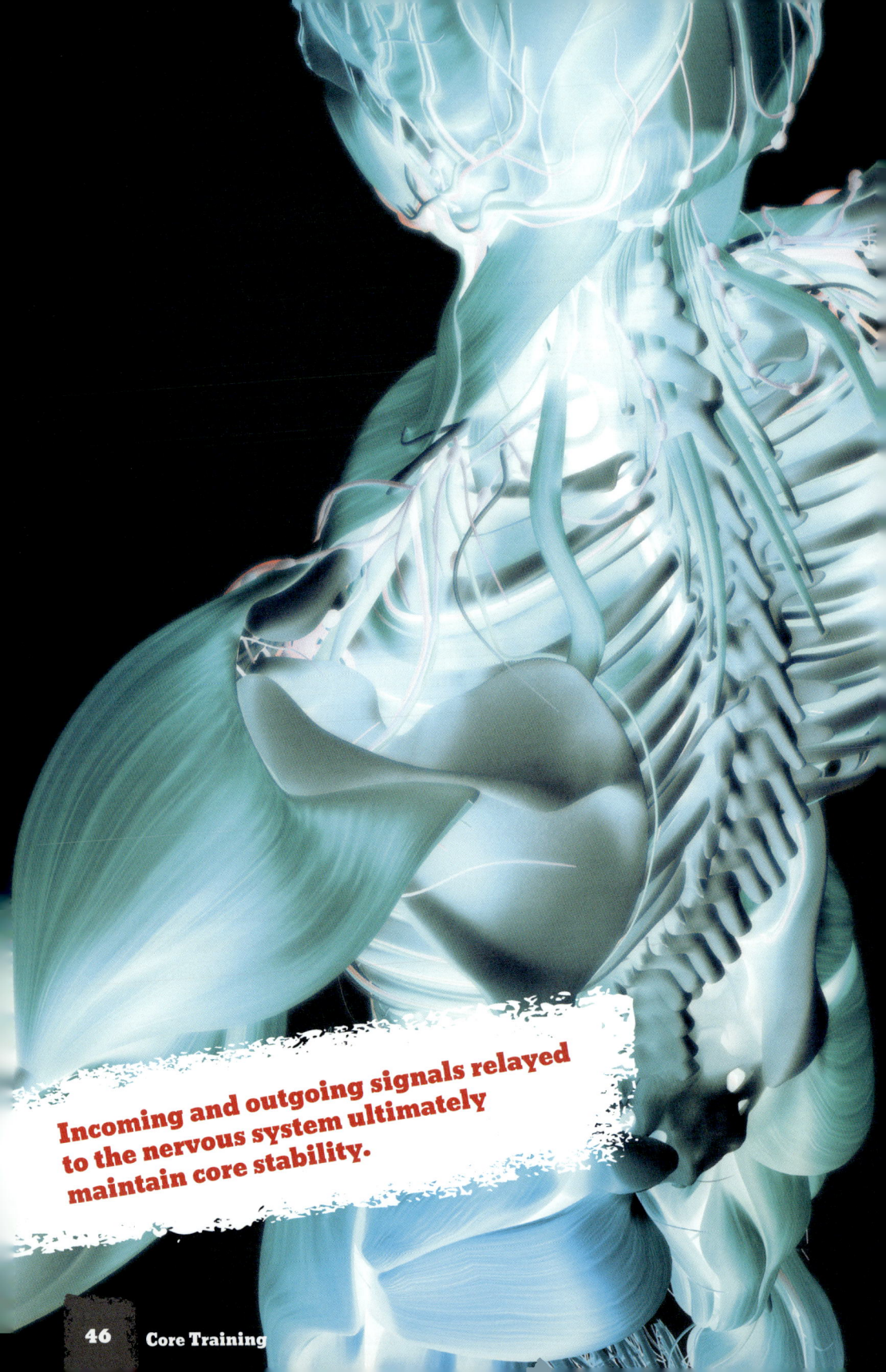

Anticipatory Postural Adjustments

Multiple studies show that sudden movements of the extremities are preceded by core activation. For example, right before you lift your arm overhead, your diaphragm, transverse abdominis (TVA), multifidus, and pelvic floor contract. These four muscles, aka the "inner core," have a unique ability to anticipate movement, activating in advance to control posture. How is this possible?

Research shows that changes in postural control are enhanced through experience. At some point during our growth and development, we received feedback from the environment about how to keep our center of mass stable. Over time, our CNS learned the exact signals to send—which muscles to contract with how much amplitude to stabilize our position. Eventually, these patterns became so ingrained that our CNS started to do them *before* movement in anticipation of instability.

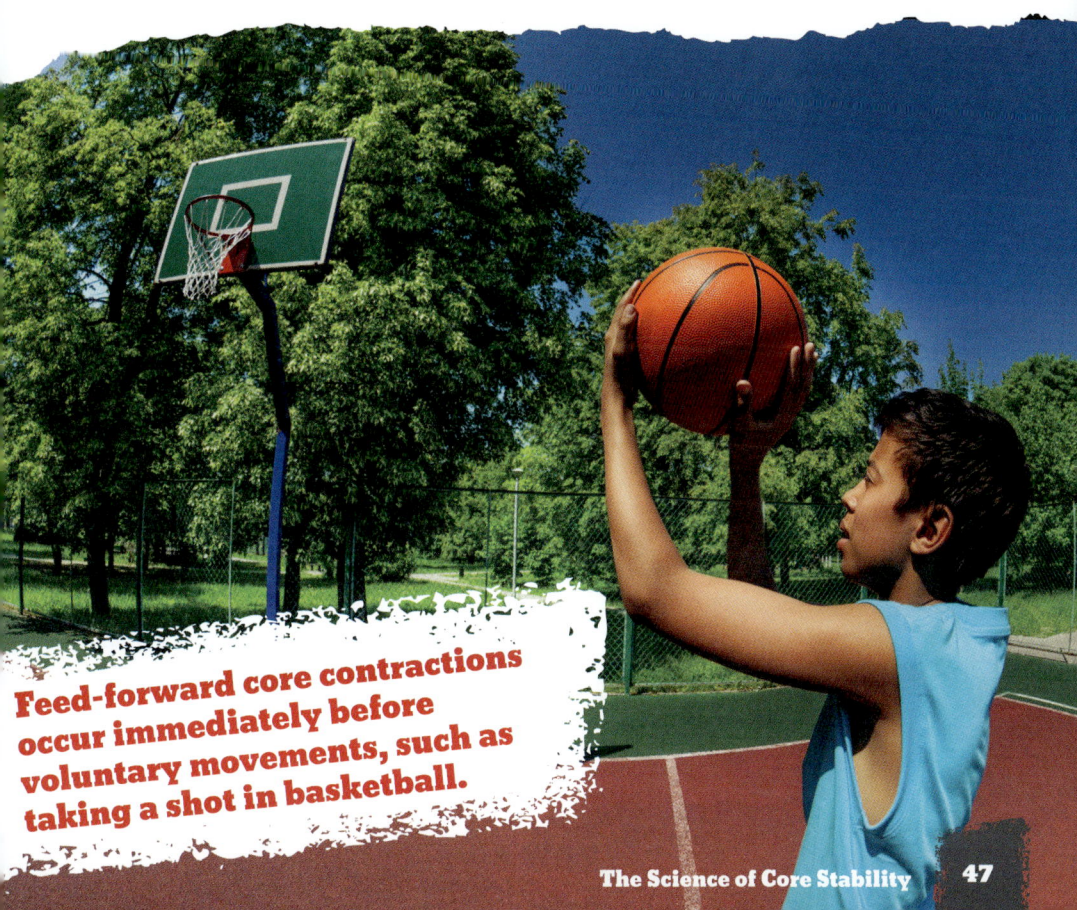

Feed-forward core contractions occur immediately before voluntary movements, such as taking a shot in basketball.

Anticipatory postural adjustments, therefore, are inner core musculature activations that come before voluntary movement. When you decide to move, a pattern of signals is sent from the brain to your muscles. Feed-forward contractions of the core occur first in an effort to reduce instability and provide a solid base. Then, nanoseconds later, you take a step, throw a ball, or initiate whatever the intended movement was. The more difficult the movement is, the stronger the preparation. Studies show that the CNS adjusts the amplitude of anticipatory contractions depending on the bodily support, how specific the task is, and distance of movement.

Reactionary Postural Adjustments

In contrast, with entirely new movements, your brain might anticipate wrong. Given that it has no frame of reference, it'll simply do its best. Novel exercises often induce instability at first, but then your "outer core" has an opportunity to react. These muscles, such as the rectus abdominis, internal and external obliques, and glutes, get input about their position in space through sensory receptors. These receptors transmit information to the brain through **afferent neurons** or sensory neurons that carry impulses away from the muscles to the CNS. Your brain processes that information, decides what to do, and sends a message back to the muscles through **efferent neurons.** These motor

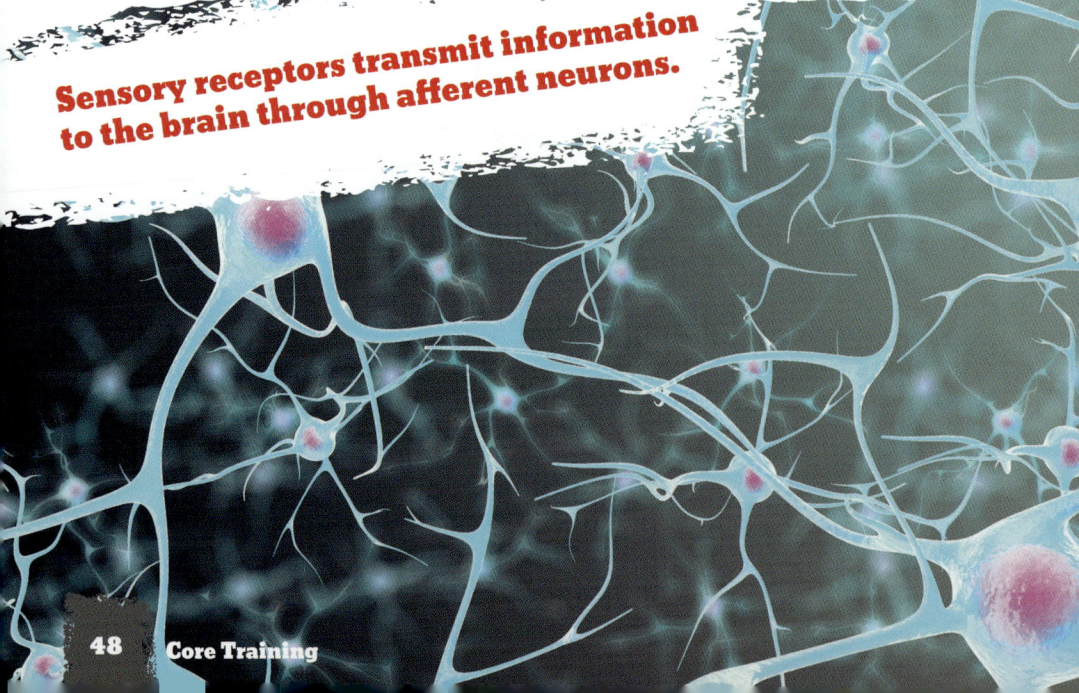

Sensory receptors transmit information to the brain through afferent neurons.

neurons trigger the appropriate muscle contraction to restabilize positioning. These interactions continue until stability is no longer required or until the outer core muscles fatigue.

Stability, Strength, and Endurance

Stability and postural control are ultimately governed by muscular contraction. The stronger and more resilient to fatigue your muscles are, the higher is their capacity to resist movement. It's a two-way street.

While your anticipatory muscles can only get so strong, the more you train them to contract before movement the less work your outer core will have to do. That's why it's important to train healthy positioning in less challenging postural conditions first. If you can teach your TVA to kick in while lying supine and moving your legs, then it'll be more likely to repeat this pattern while crawling, sitting, or standing.

Eventually, however, your anticipatory activity only goes so far. Increasing load, decreasing base of support, or adding time challenges your outer core. And just like any other muscle, training it in the gym makes it

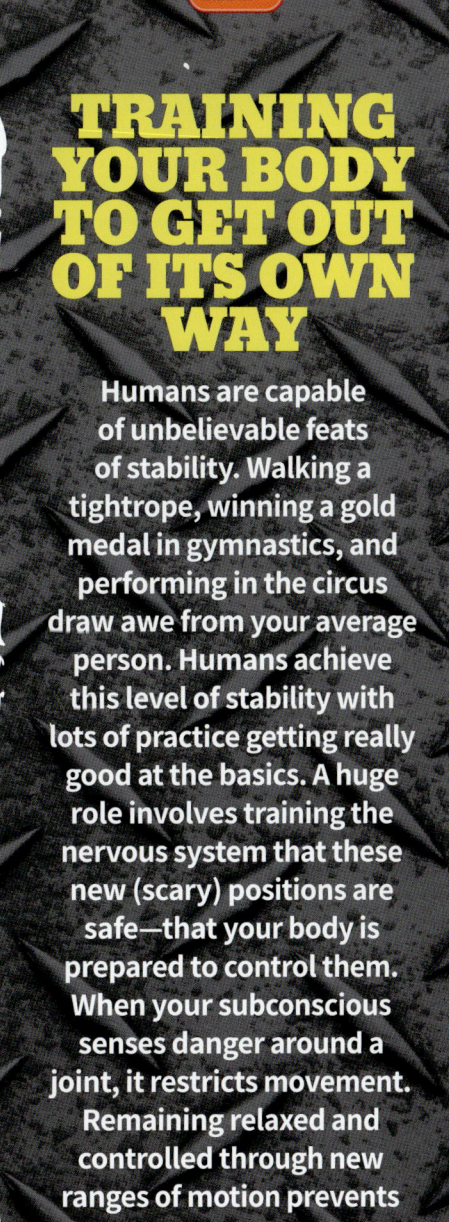

TRAINING YOUR BODY TO GET OUT OF ITS OWN WAY

Humans are capable of unbelievable feats of stability. Walking a tightrope, winning a gold medal in gymnastics, and performing in the circus draw awe from your average person. Humans achieve this level of stability with lots of practice getting really good at the basics. A huge role involves training the nervous system that these new (scary) positions are safe—that your body is prepared to control them. When your subconscious senses danger around a joint, it restricts movement. Remaining relaxed and controlled through new ranges of motion prevents reflexive tightening. The key to elite athleticism is training stability and movement as one.

 Training like a Cirque du Soleil performer involves remaining relaxed and controlled through the range of movements.

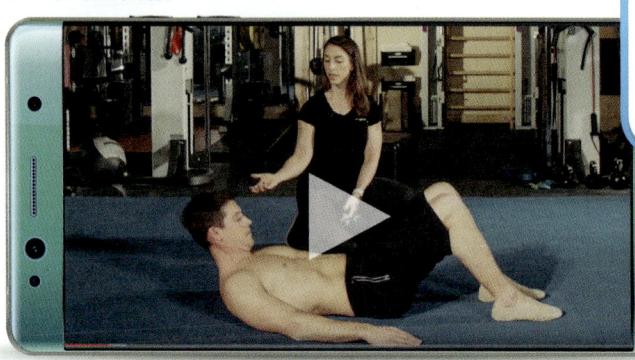

Core muscles such as the glutes, rectus femoris, and iliopsoas as well as the adductors, lats, and pecs are responsible for transferring force along the kinetic chain.

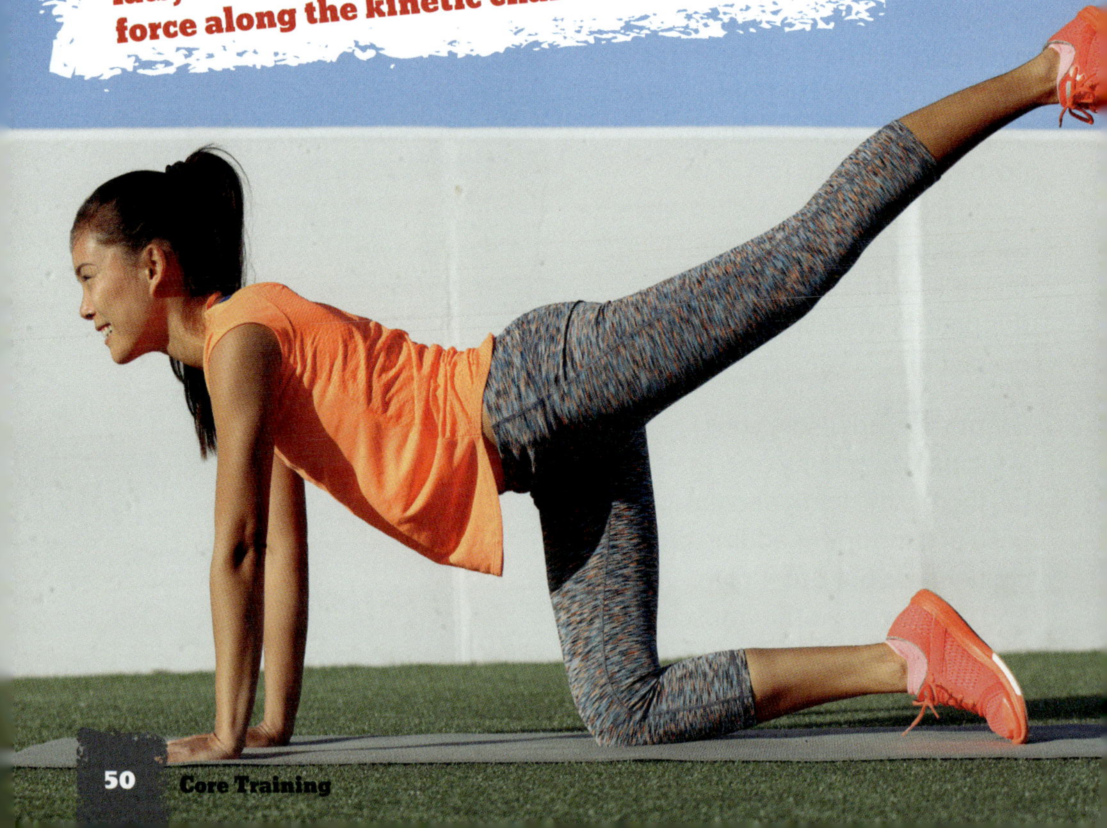

stronger. Core stability training, therefore, grooves neuronal patterns, improves localized muscular endurance, and trains load transfer.

Load Transfer Muscles

Muscles that attach the extremities to your torso, including core muscles such as the glutes, rectus femoris, and iliopsoas as well as the adductors, lats, and pecs are responsible for transferring force along the kinetic chain. As these muscles cover multiple joints, their activation controls complex patterns of movement. Successful transfer of load requires initial stability on one side of a joint and motion on the other. As energy is generated along one point of the chain, contraction of the load transfer muscles gathers that force, redirects it, and expresses it at the chain's end. While we know this force distribution occurs, surprisingly little is understood as to how it works. Regardless, strengthening neuromuscular patterning as well as the contractile ability and stiffness of these muscles can improve power transfer.

TEXT-DEPENDENT QUESTIONS

1. What roles do core stability and mobility have in load transfer across the kinetic chain?

2. Name three factors that affect how the CNS adjusts the amplitude of anticipatory contractions.

3. Why is breathing with your diaphragm crucial to optimal core stability?

RESEARCH PROJECT

Pick the single-leg squat, push-up, or squat jump and trace the actions of core stability from start to finish. Include which muscles are being worked, the neuronal signals, and the role of positioning in execution.

WORDS TO UNDERSTAND

kinetic energy—the energy something possesses by virtue of being in motion

movement economy—the energy required to maintain a constant velocity of movement. With greater movement economy comes greater efficiency

torque—a twisting force caused by rotation around an axis

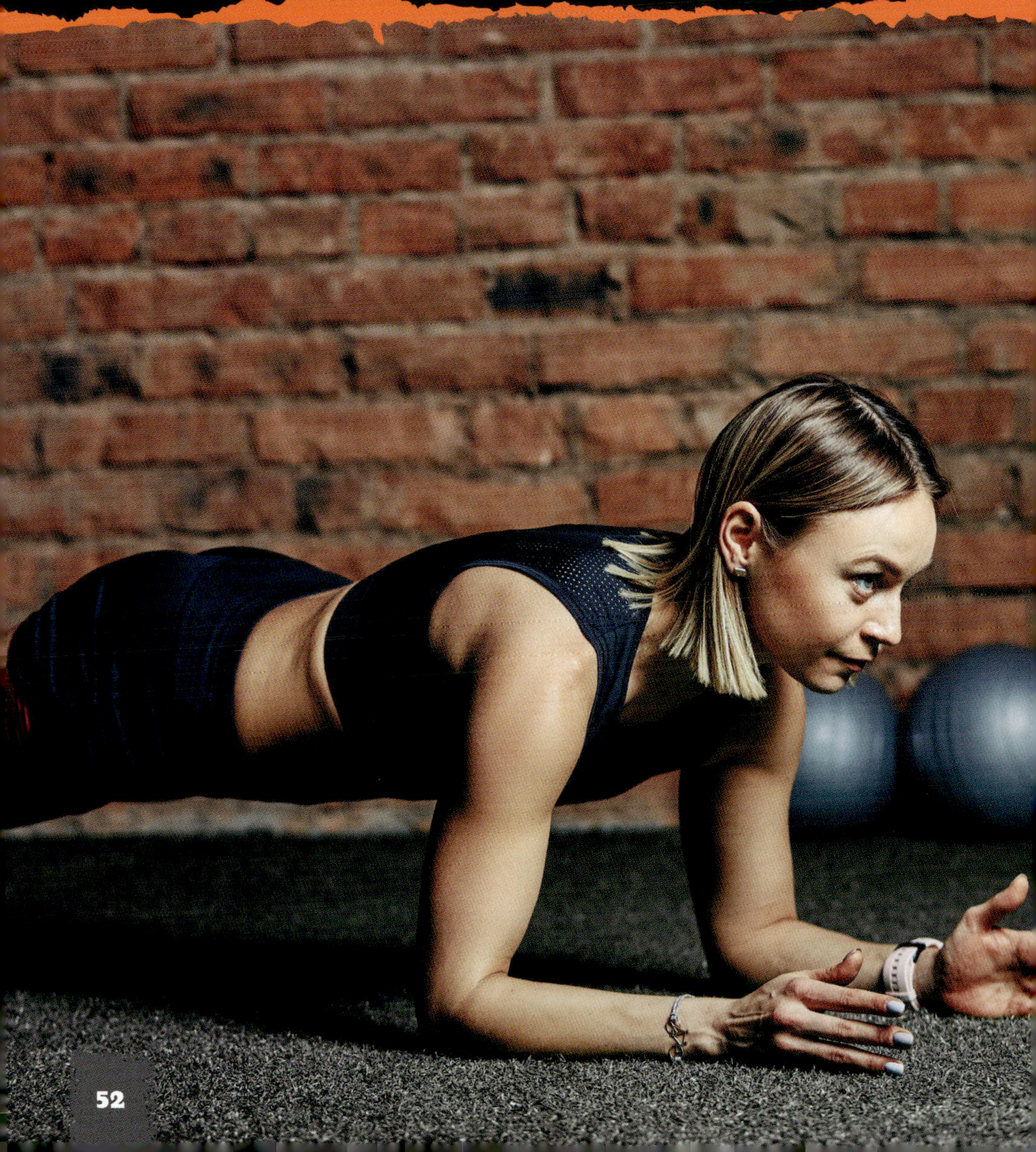

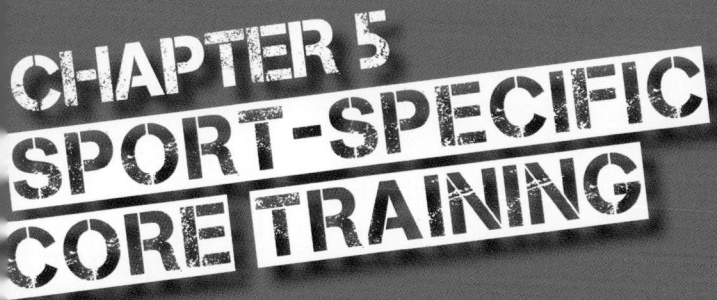

CHAPTER 5
SPORT-SPECIFIC CORE TRAINING

GENERAL ATHLETICISM

Athleticism is such a broad term, considering the wide array of sports and physical activities. According to the late Bob Singer, former head of the University of Florida Department of Exercise and Sports Sciences, motor performance can be defined along scales of accuracy, force, velocity, and reaction time. Training a specific task repeatedly, therefore, improves performance through learning. As core training for athleticism requires repeating sport-specific movements—a majority of which will occur in practice and competition.

In order to achieve optimum athletic ability, however, you need a strong base of support, precision, and power. A smart approach to sport-specific core training, therefore, would be first to control stability and then train the body to avoid "energy leaks" along the kinetic chain.

Four key areas of sport-specific core training include:

> Local and global postural control
> Positional bracing
> Power transfer
> Deceleration

Local and Global Postural Control

Athletes need to train their cores to anticipate changes in center of mass or common voluntary movements. For example, throwers (i.e., quarterbacks and pitchers) should train core stability with arms overhead to maximize potential force output. As mentioned in previous chapters, these local and global systems work in tandem to withstand disturbances in motion. These neuromuscular responses can be trained with low-level bracing exercise activity, such as plank variations, dead bugs, and bear crawls.

Positional Bracing

As neuromuscular patterns become enhanced with practice, it's important to train in sport-specific positions. Most sports involve standing up, so effective core training takes place while upright. Outside of power transfer, the core's primary role in sports is bracing against limb movement or external force. Therefore, exercises such as Pallof presses, rotational lunges, and weighted carries provide more transfer to competition.

Power Transfer

To tackle, sprint, and throw, power travels from the legs through the core, propelling an athlete's upper body through space. Before any of this can happen, however, we have to create force. Whether it's driving our feet into the floor or generating rotational **torque**, our legs play a huge role. Strengthen the legs first and then focus on maintaining that force. The skill and timing of sport-specific movements warrant core training focused on optimizing technique. For example, throwers need to throw and jumpers should jump. All core training for power transfer should be done with a low to moderate level of added resistance (i.e., resistance bands, medicine balls, weight vests, etc.).

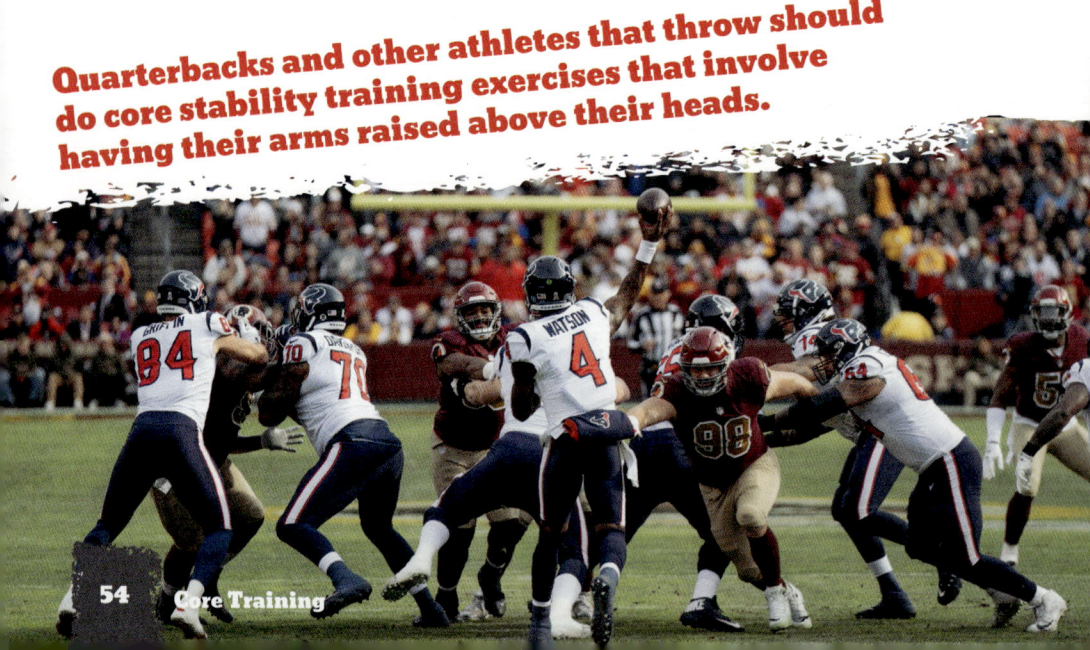

Quarterbacks and other athletes that throw should do core stability training exercises that involve having their arms raised above their heads.

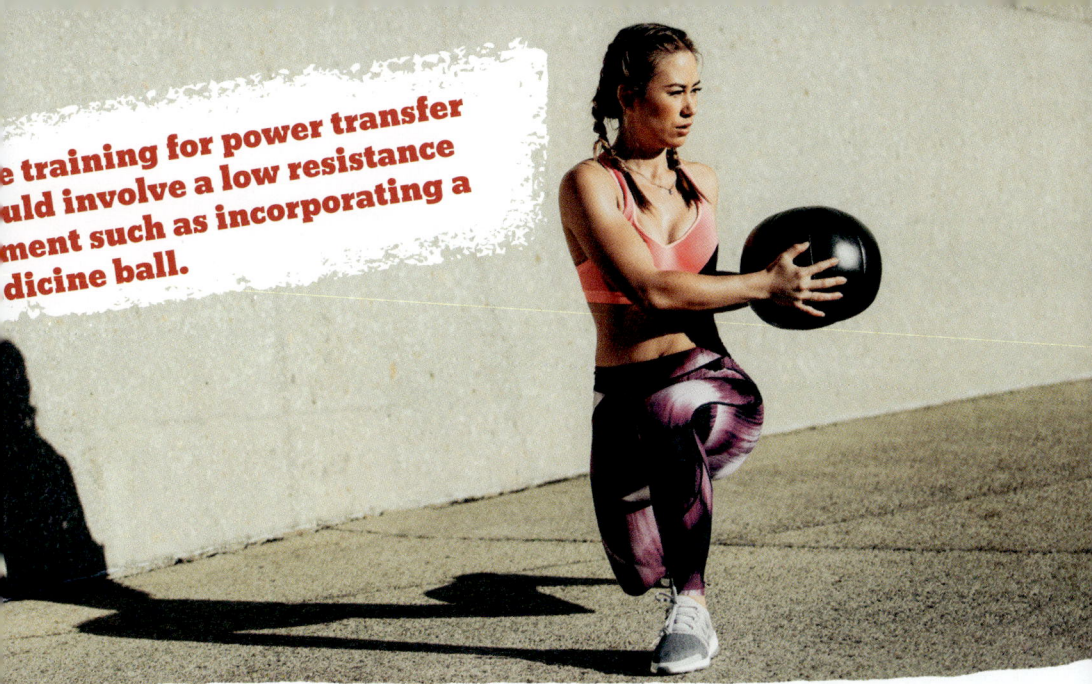

...e training for power transfer ...uld involve a low resistance ...ment such as incorporating a ...dicine ball.

Deceleration

Coaches and athletes love to talk about how fast you can move, but how fast can you stop? Deceleration helps change direction on a dime, evade defenders, and break down just before a shot. It's also the primary mechanism behind injury prevention. Antagonist muscles slow down force to prevent damage to the joints. Without deceleration, our legs would fly off every time we tried to kick a ball. The core plays a massive role in containing that force, pulling us back into a safe range of motion.

CORE TRAINING FOR NON-CONTACT TEAM SPORTS

Sports such as basketball, soccer, lacrosse, and hockey all require quick changes of direction. They're a mix of endurance, power, and skill, and they all involve controlling an external object, whether that is a ball, stick, or another implement. Therefore, these sports require elite levels of coordination. Athletes need enough stiffness to transfer and absorb force, yet enough mobility to sprint past defenders. By reverse-engineering the demands of the sport, we can isolate the core.

As all of these sports take place while upright, start with the single-leg Y-balance test to assess dynamic stability. Begin balancing on

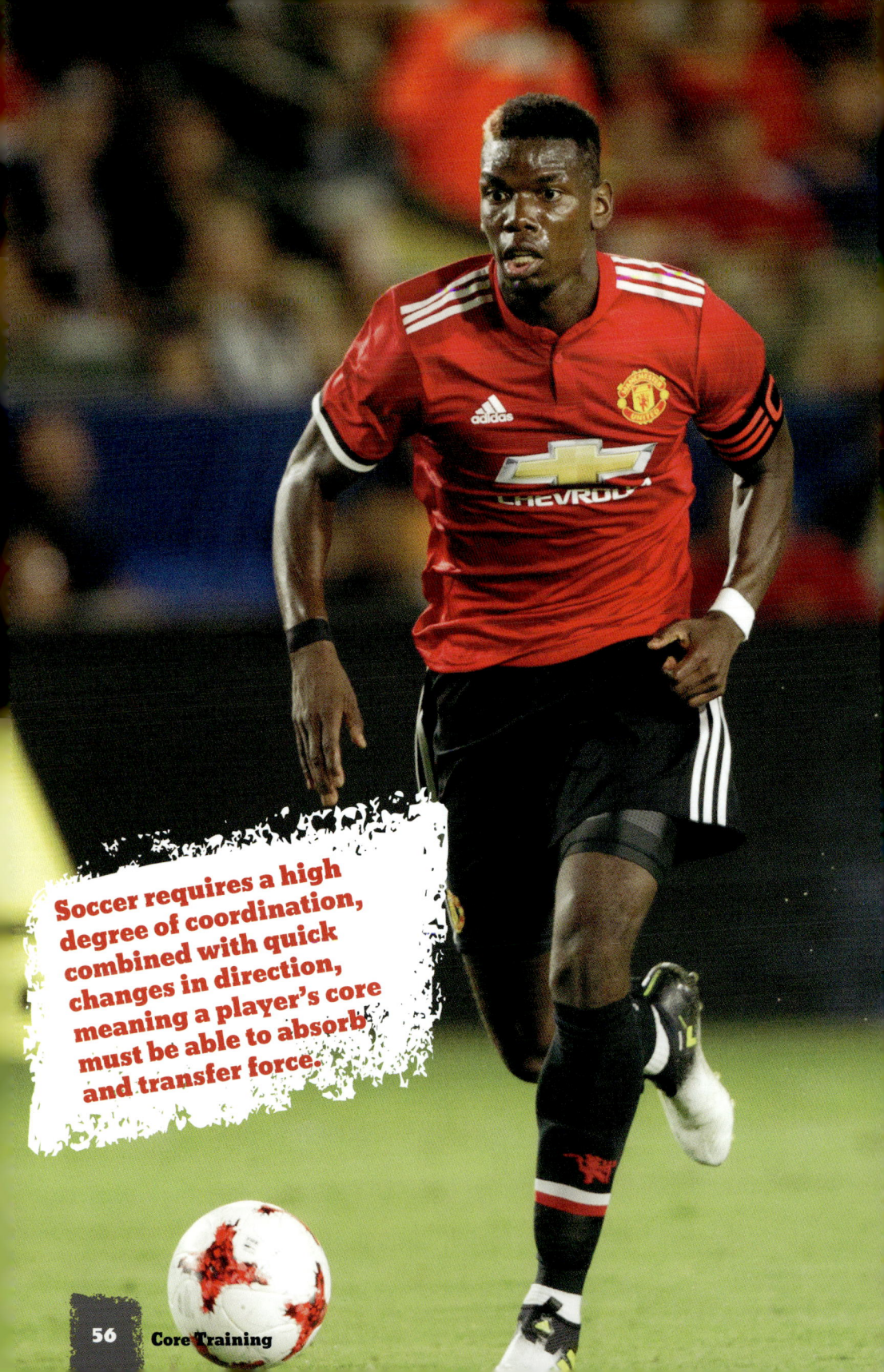

Soccer requires a high degree of coordination, combined with quick changes in direction, meaning a player's core must be able to absorb and transfer force.

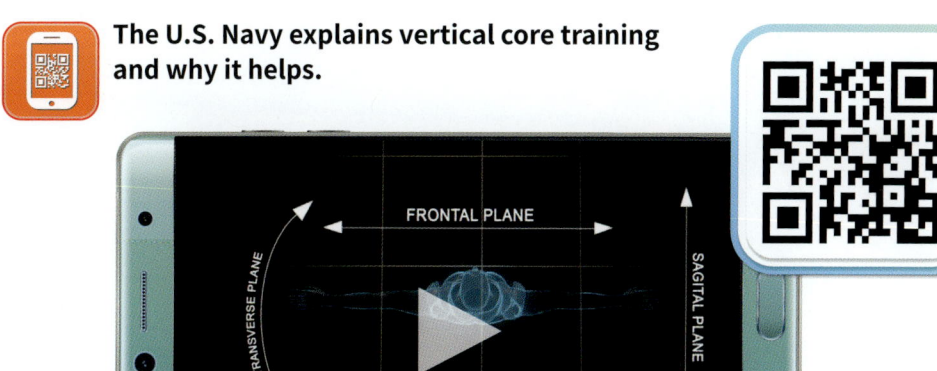

The U.S. Navy explains vertical core training and why it helps.

one leg and stretch the other leg forward, backward to the left, and backward to the right (as if you're attempting to draw a "Y" with your foot). When used as a movement screen, this test correlated with the likelihood of lower extremity injury in Division I college athletes. The farther an athlete could reach without deviating or falling over, the less likely they were to get hurt. First train your single-leg balance to score well on this test and then move on to more dynamic methods.

On top of general core development, non-contact team sport athletes should focus on exercises that mimic their sport. While a majority of core training will come from practice itself, use any form of vertical loading, producing, or resisting directional force in the gym. Examples include weighted throws, resisted rotation, single-leg bounds, sprinting, and deceleration.

ENDURANCE SPORTS

Running, swimming, cycling, and other endurance sports challenge the core's ability to sustain posture. Therefore, core endurance is the most critical component of training for these sports. As the extremities are in constant motion, the muscles of the core react accordingly to maintain stability. Keeping the trunk and pelvis in the ideal position could make the difference between winning a race and getting injured.

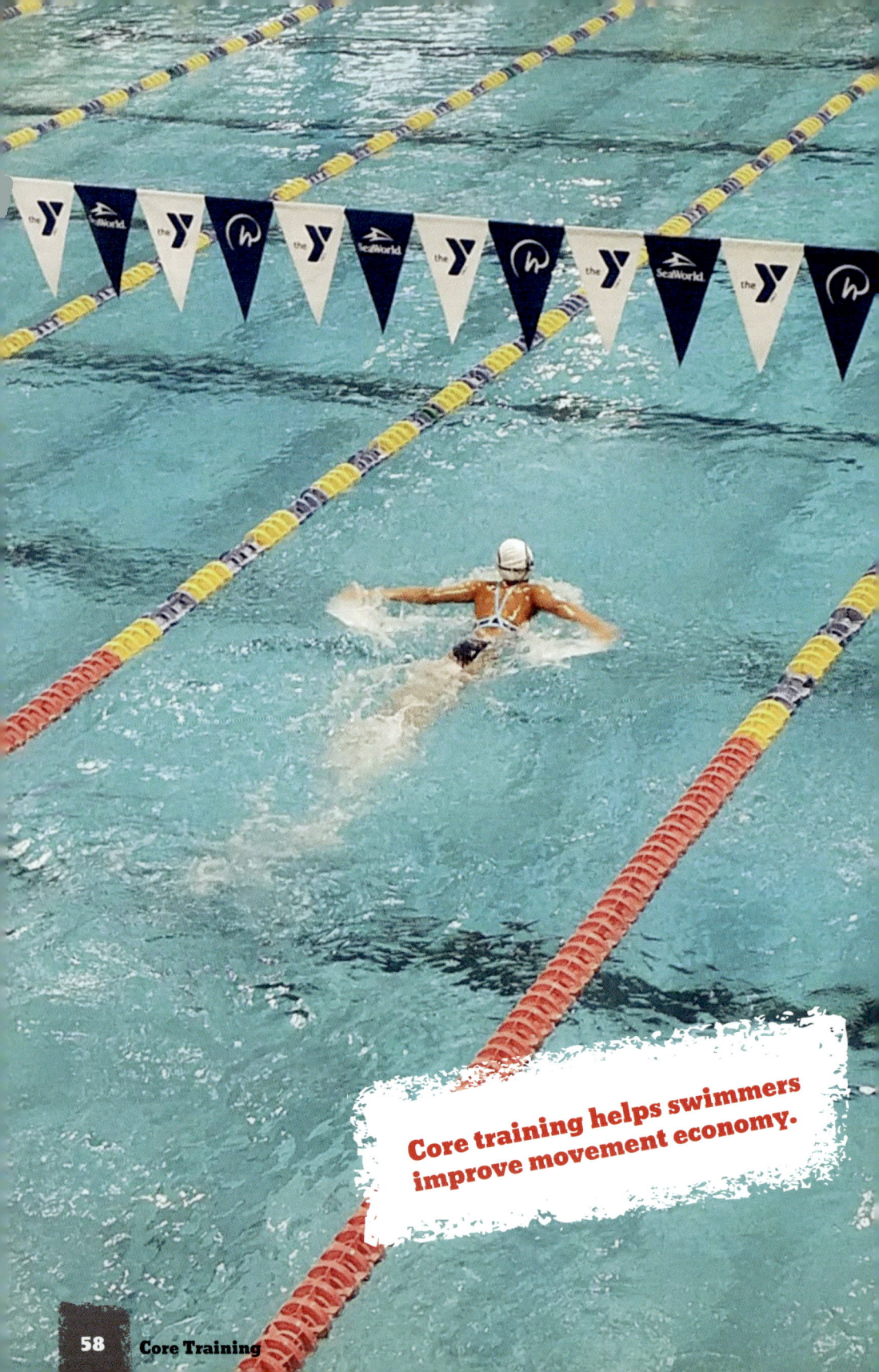

Core training helps swimmers improve movement economy.

Core training for these sports can improve **movement economy**, reducing a loss of power in each step or stroke. When researchers looked at collegiate athletes, they found that eight weeks of core training improved running economy, balance, and endurance. Functional training suggests anti-movement exercises, such as resisting rotation, extension, or flexion, to maintain trunk positioning while using one's extremities. Start with exercises on the ground or on all fours, such as dead bugs and bird dogs, then move to Pallof presses, carries, or lunges with resisted rotation.

POWER SPORTS

Weightlifting, throwing, sprinting, and even baseball require a huge amount of force generation and transfer. The core's role in rotation and triple extension is to transfer power from one limb to the next. A smart approach to training would be to maximize force production first and then ensure that there are no energy leaks during activity. As the majority of power comes from the hips, training the legs and glutes is key for any power athlete. Then, focus on stabilizing the pillar across the planes of motion required in the sport.

Finally, train the ability to decelerate and regenerate force. Athletes can generate a ton of torque by twisting their body like a spring. In sports, a lot of **kinetic energy** gets absorbed by passive tissue and then redirected in the desired direction. For example, baseball players can benefit from catching, stopping, and hurdling a medicine ball with one hand. As each power movement is highly coordinated, train at the speeds and angles you experience in competition. Break an entire throw, sprint, or lift into pieces, work on the components individually, and then string them together. Start with deceleration core work, then concentric only, and finally combine both.

CONTACT SPORTS

In contact sports such as football, rugby, wrestling, and martial arts, athletes are constantly moving/resisting other people's bodies. They require strength and power in odd positions, crouched over to make a tackle or on one's back trying to wrestle from the bottom. The best core training comes from practicing your sport under controlled

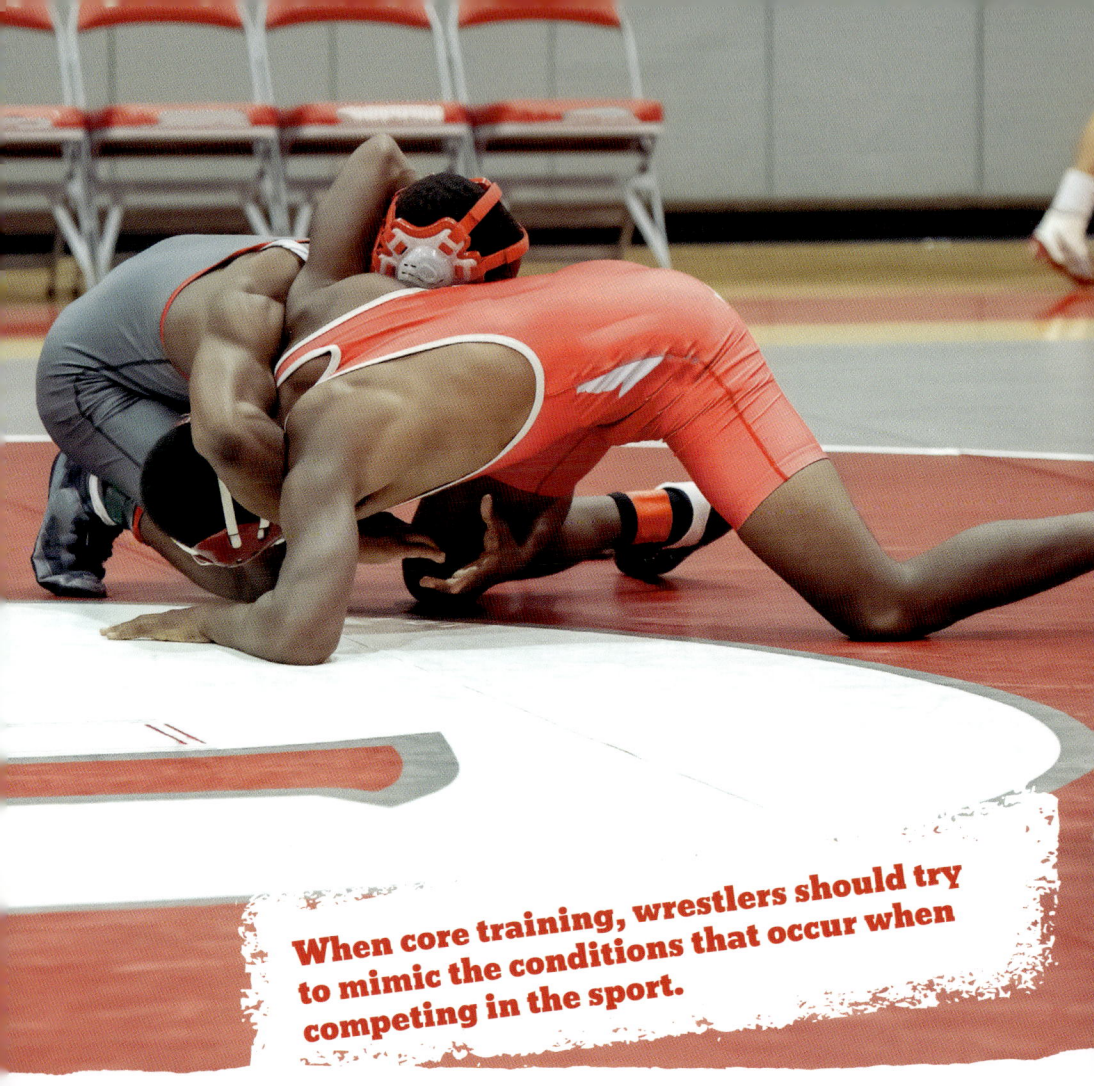

When core training, wrestlers should try to mimic the conditions that occur when competing in the sport.

circumstances. For example, rugby players can get on all fours in a bear crawl position while a partner attempts to roll them over. Wrestlers can fight against holds to scramble out and stand up. Football players can rip and roll defenders to break through tackles.

Gym-based core training should be focused primarily on injury prevention. In contact sports, unlike most other sports, the arms and legs are likely to end up locked in place during force production. This means workouts should strengthen the extremities through full range of motion, primarily focusing on stability of the shoulder and hip. Exercises that lock the legs while moving the arms (or vice versa), including planks with reaches and rotations, Pallof presses, windshield wipers, and hanging leg raises, are beneficial. Training should also feature carrying and controlling odd objects, such as maces, sandbags, or sleds.

TRICK-BASED SPORTS

Gymnastics, diving, extreme sports, figure skating, and other trick-based sports require an extreme level of body control. Core training for these sports, therefore, should primarily focus on manipulating one's body through space. Ultimately, the stronger one's core, the better control these athletes will have. Planks, Swiss ball pikes, windshield wipers, toes-to-bar, and others all set a solid foundation. After establishing adequate control and stability (think ~2–3-minute holds, 20+ reps, etc.), add in sport specificity. For example, surfers and snowboarders should practice explosive rotation/anti-rotation in their competition stance. Figure out what positions require stability, which require rapid contraction, and work backward from there.

Core training and stability form a critical part of injury prevention for trick-based athletes. As the functional connection between the upper and lower body, these sports place an insane amount of stress upon the core. Therefore,

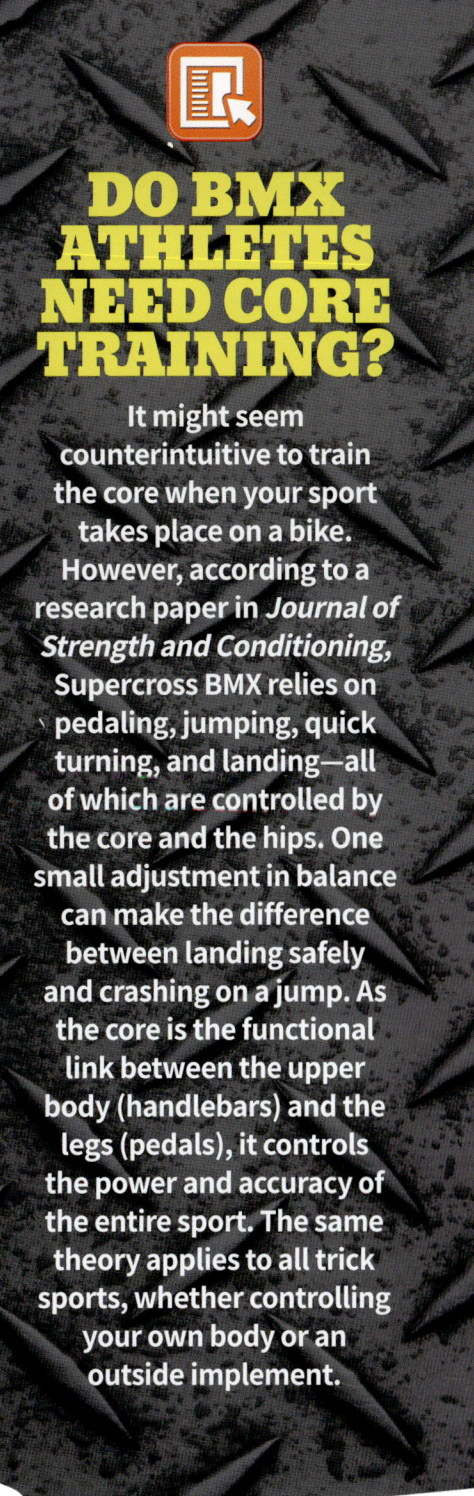

DO BMX ATHLETES NEED CORE TRAINING?

It might seem counterintuitive to train the core when your sport takes place on a bike. However, according to a research paper in *Journal of Strength and Conditioning,* Supercross BMX relies on pedaling, jumping, quick turning, and landing—all of which are controlled by the core and the hips. One small adjustment in balance can make the difference between landing safely and crashing on a jump. As the core is the functional link between the upper body (handlebars) and the legs (pedals), it controls the power and accuracy of the entire sport. The same theory applies to all trick sports, whether controlling your own body or an outside implement.

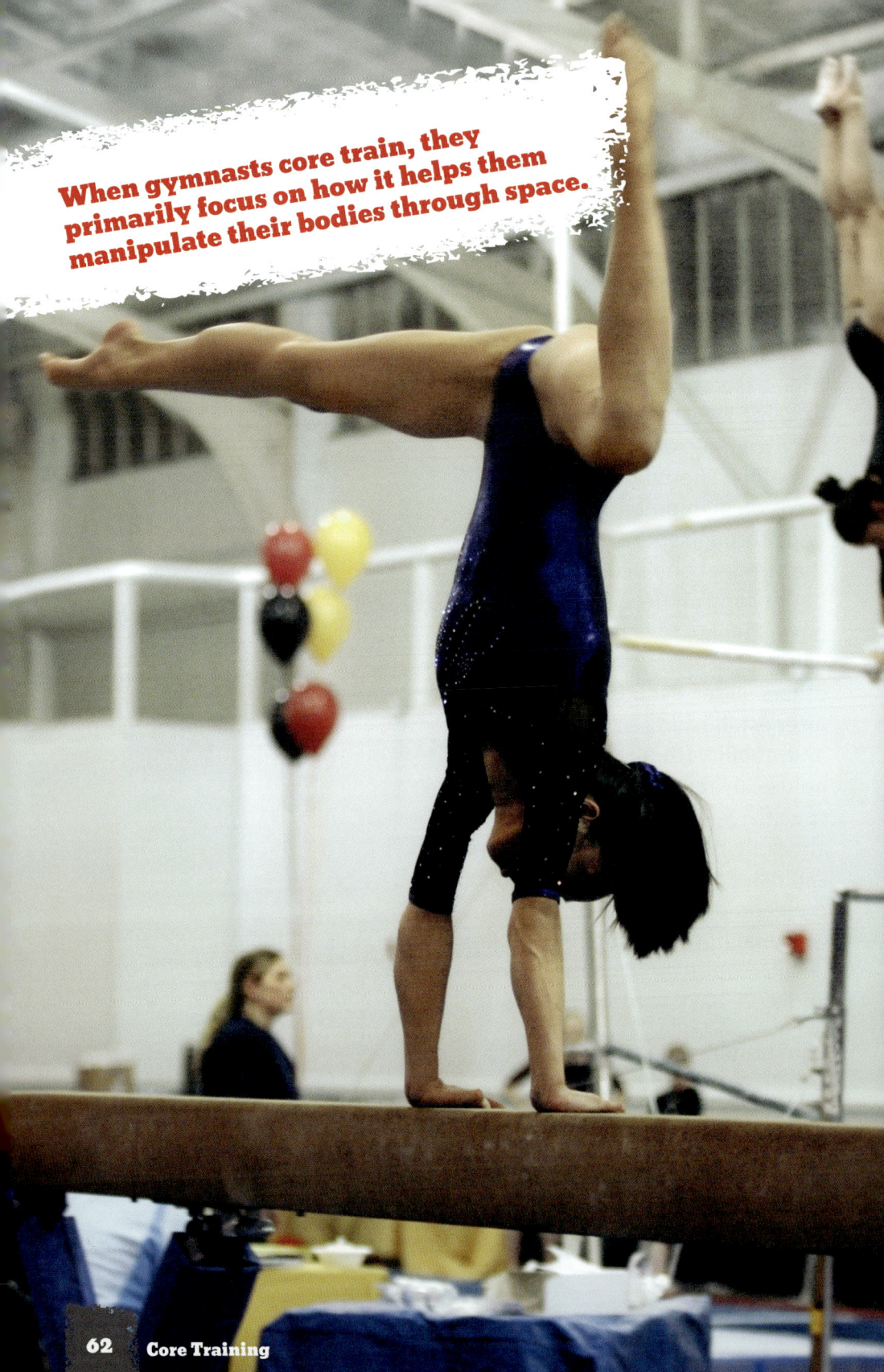

When gymnasts core train, they primarily focus on how it helps them manipulate their bodies through space.

a well-rounded program to develop core endurance is paramount. When researchers looked at the effects of fatigue on trunk stability in gymnasts, they found that it was much more difficult for tired athletes to stay balanced. Fatigue induced by a realistic training load decreases stability, which makes athletes more susceptible to falls, missteps, and injury. To lessen the injury risk, they should incorporate progressive core training daily across all planes of movement.

TEXT-DEPENDENT QUESTIONS

1. While all sports require it to some degree, which type of sport relies *most* heavily on the core's ability to transfer energy? Why?
2. Identify the importance of core endurance in distance running.
3. If sports are dynamic and constantly changing, why are postural control and bracing critical to elite sports performance?

RESEARCH PROJECT

Choose your favorite sport and design a core workout for an athlete competing in that sport. Make sure to include 5–10 exercises that optimize both sports performance and injury prevention.

WORDS TO UNDERSTAND

non-specific lower back pain—refers to uncomfortable or painful symptoms without a specific cause
proprioception—the awareness of our body's position and movement in space
specific lower back pain—involves a clearly identifiable cause, such as disk injury from a car accident or muscle strain

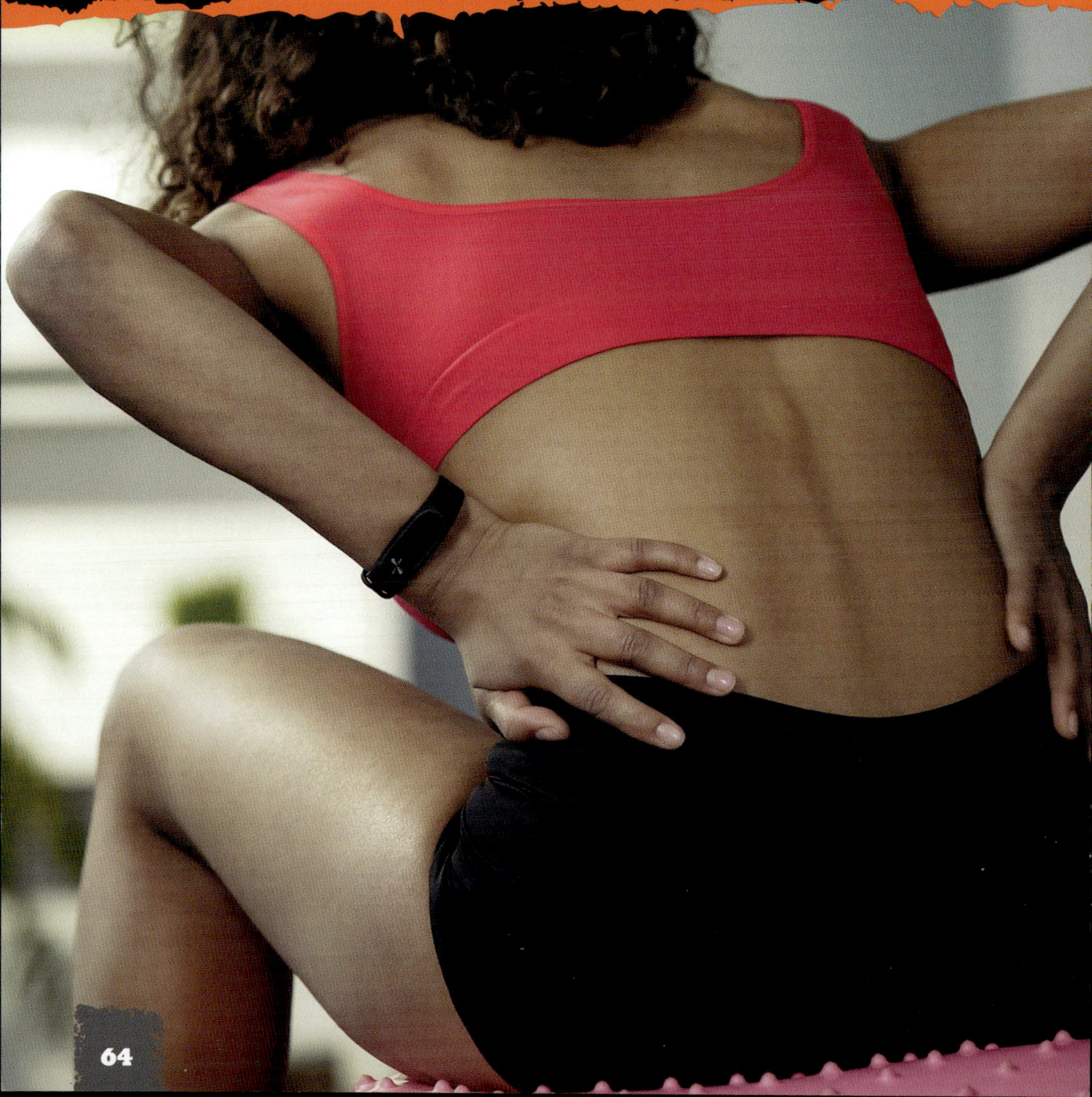

Chapter 6
Common Injuries: How Core Training Prevents Them

According to *International Journal of Sports Physical Therapy,* a lack of core stability is associated with upper extremity, lower back, and lower limb injuries. Despite a "gold-standard" assessment, core training remains a vital component of injury prevention and rehabilitation. Strengthening the core helps limit fatigue, correct for errors in movement, and resist joint damage.

A comprehensive training program starts with fine-tuning the local neuromuscular control of the muscles that stabilize the core. Once that's been established, athletes can progress to exercises challenging the stability of global stabilizers as well. Finally, core training should include dynamic functional movements, requiring one to maintain the first two aspects. Functional movement screens can be used to determine how a person ranks among these aspects of core stability and exercises should be chosen accordingly.

Examples for neuromuscular control exercises:

> Diaphragmatic breathing
> Pelvic tilt control
> Hollow body holds
> Abdominal bracing

Examples for stabilization exercises:

> Bird dogs
> Dead bugs
> Front plank
> Side plank

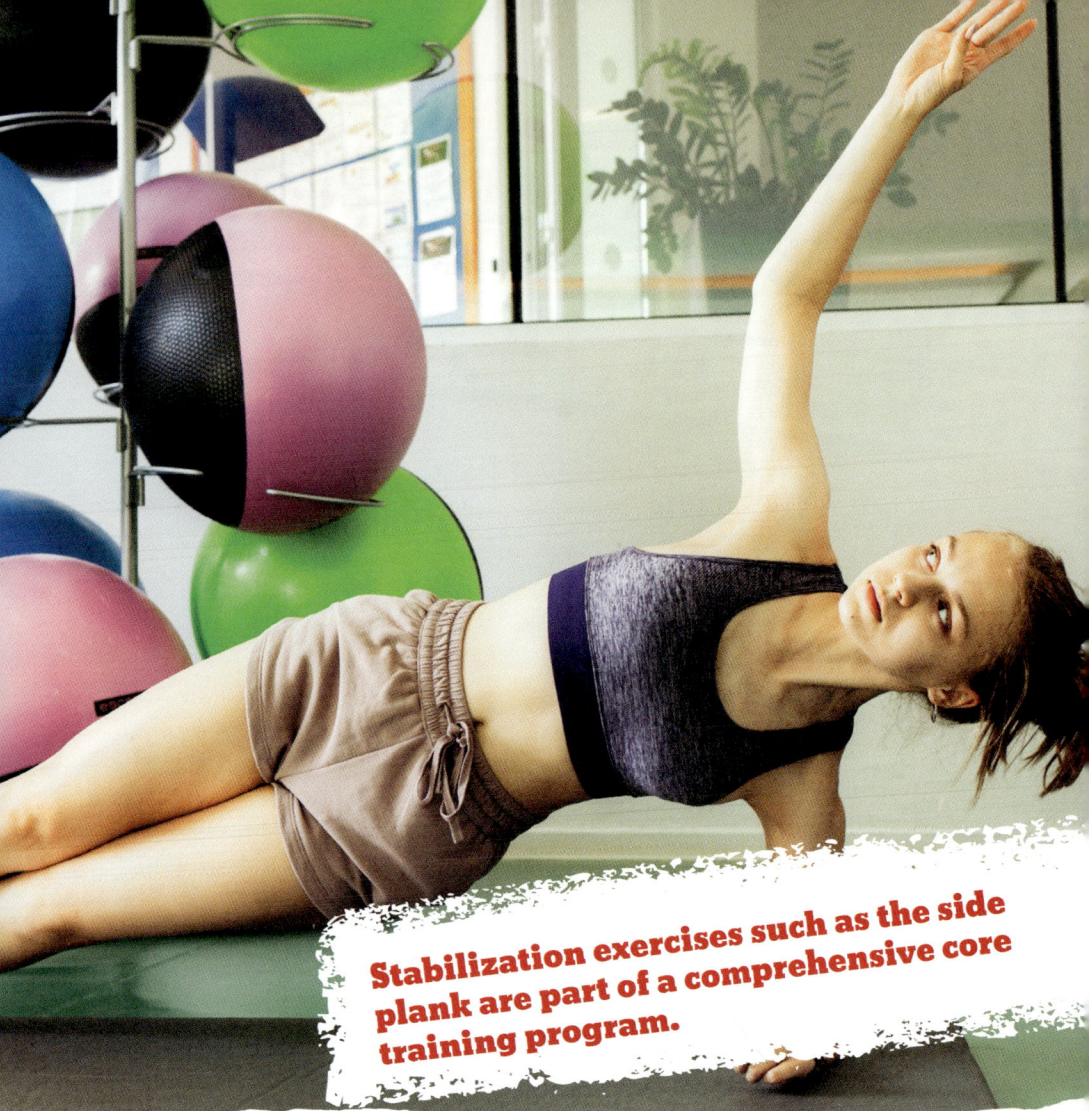

Stabilization exercises such as the side plank are part of a comprehensive core training program.

Examples for dynamic functional movements:

> - Jumping and landing
> - Lunging
> - Plyometric throws
> - Single-leg balance
> - Bear crawls

LOW BACK PAIN

Millions of people deal with lower back pain every year. From acute strains to tight muscles, it's an injury that plagues almost everyone at

 Learn how to train the core to help prevent lower back injury.

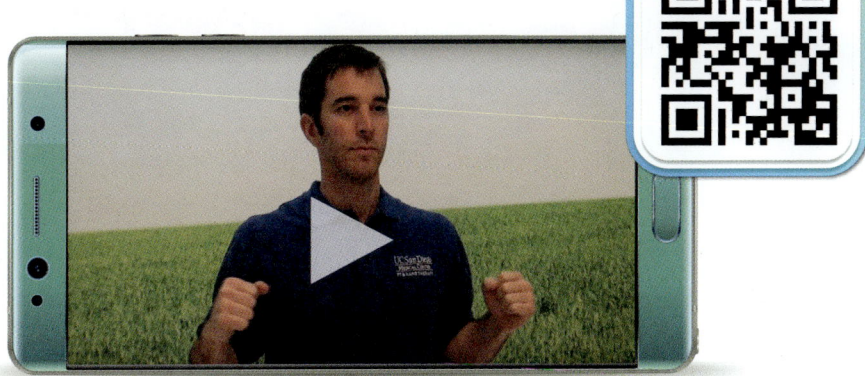

some point. As part of the core, lower back muscles often end up on one extreme of the spectrum—carrying too much or too little of the load.

According to research published by Marienke van Middelkoop et al. in 2010, lower back pain can be divided between specific and nonspecific types. **Specific lower back pain** involves a clearly identifiable cause, such as disk injury from a car accident or muscle strain. This type of pain results from traumatic loading or degeneration, which can be prevented via core training. **Non-specific lower back pain** refers to uncomfortable or painful symptoms without a specific cause. As it's unclear what causes non-specific pain, it's impossible to prescribe a solution that works in every case. However, experts suggest that a relationship may exist between exercise levels, sports participation, age, and body mass index. Regardless, we know that a lack of core strength contributes negatively to the coordination of muscles that protect the lumbar spine, increasing the risk of both specific and non-specific injury.

Developing well-rounded core strength and stability can ease the pressure on muscles like the quadratus lumborum and erectors. Weak glutes and a tight iliopsoas often go hand-in-hand, leading to uncomfortable pelvic tilt. Over time, this inefficient positioning wears down on joints, muscles, and connective tissue. It's like constantly bending and pulling at a small fray on a cord. Eventually, things start to break down.

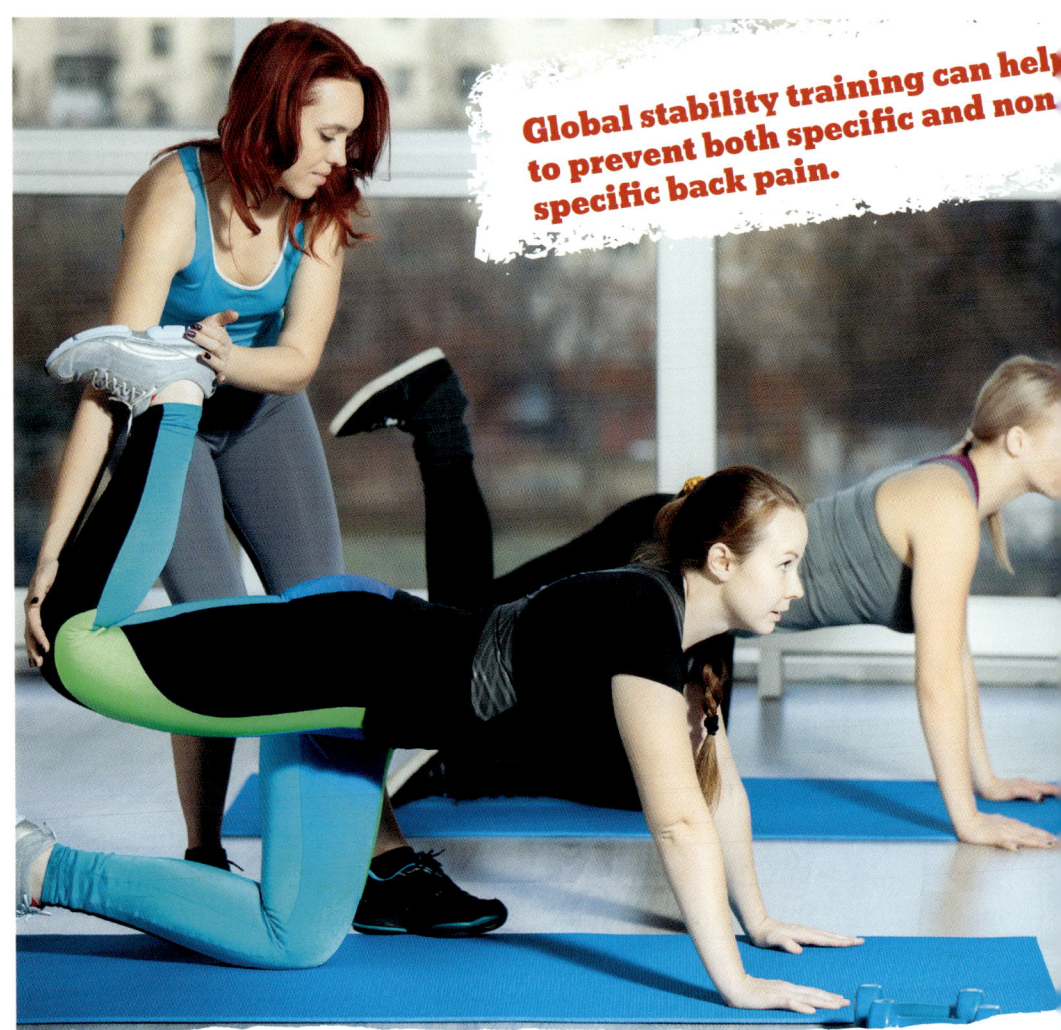

Global stability training can help to prevent both specific and non-specific back pain.

Decreased trunk and hip extensor endurance can even predict future cases of low back pain. When researchers tested the static back endurance of non-athletes through the Trunk Extensor Test, a lack of strength was the only physical predictor of pain. In athletes, a delayed reflexive response of abdominal muscles increases the odds of sustaining a lower back injury. Identified as pre-existing risk factors, implementing local endurance and global stability training could prevent specific and non-specific back pain.

Research by Hodges et al. showed that local stabilizer muscles change recruitment activity in response to lower back pain, limiting their ability to stabilize the spine and relay information relating to stimuli. In healthy subjects, the transverse abdominis was recruited first, prior to movement of the extremities. This was followed by the activation of the multifidus, obliques, and rectus abdominis. In contrast, this anticipatory activation was significantly delayed in patients with lower back pain. In lower body movements, gluteus maximus activation was delayed as well, indicating one's inability to stabilize the pelvis during injury. Overall, these results suggest that deficient core stability and load transfer correlate with lower back pain.

Examples of core training to prevent back pain include:

> Plank variations
> Diaphragmatic breathing
> Pallof pressing
> Hollow body holds
> Bear crawls
> Glute bridge marches
> Clamshells

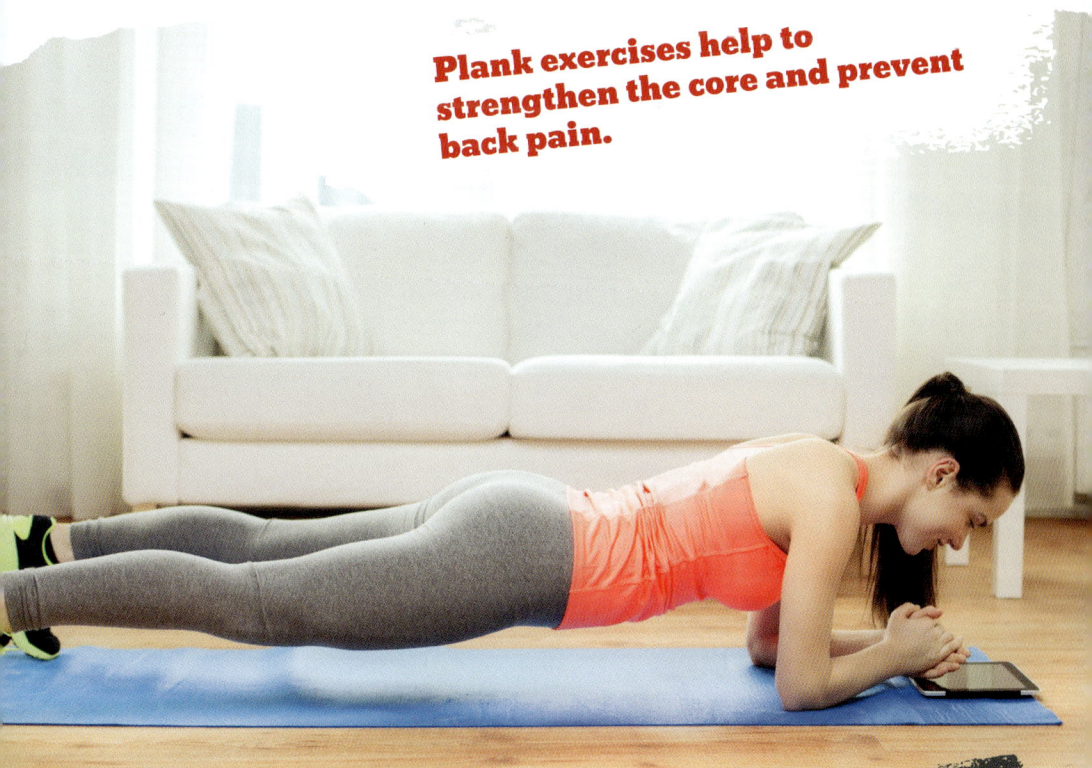

Plank exercises help to strengthen the core and prevent back pain.

KNEE INJURIES

As the knee forms the functional link between the pelvis and the ground, core stability plays a huge role in knee injury prevention. When the foot is locked in place, one wrong move puts the ligaments in the knee at risk. Therefore, healthy **proprioception**, reflexive feedback, and feed-forward mechanisms are critical.

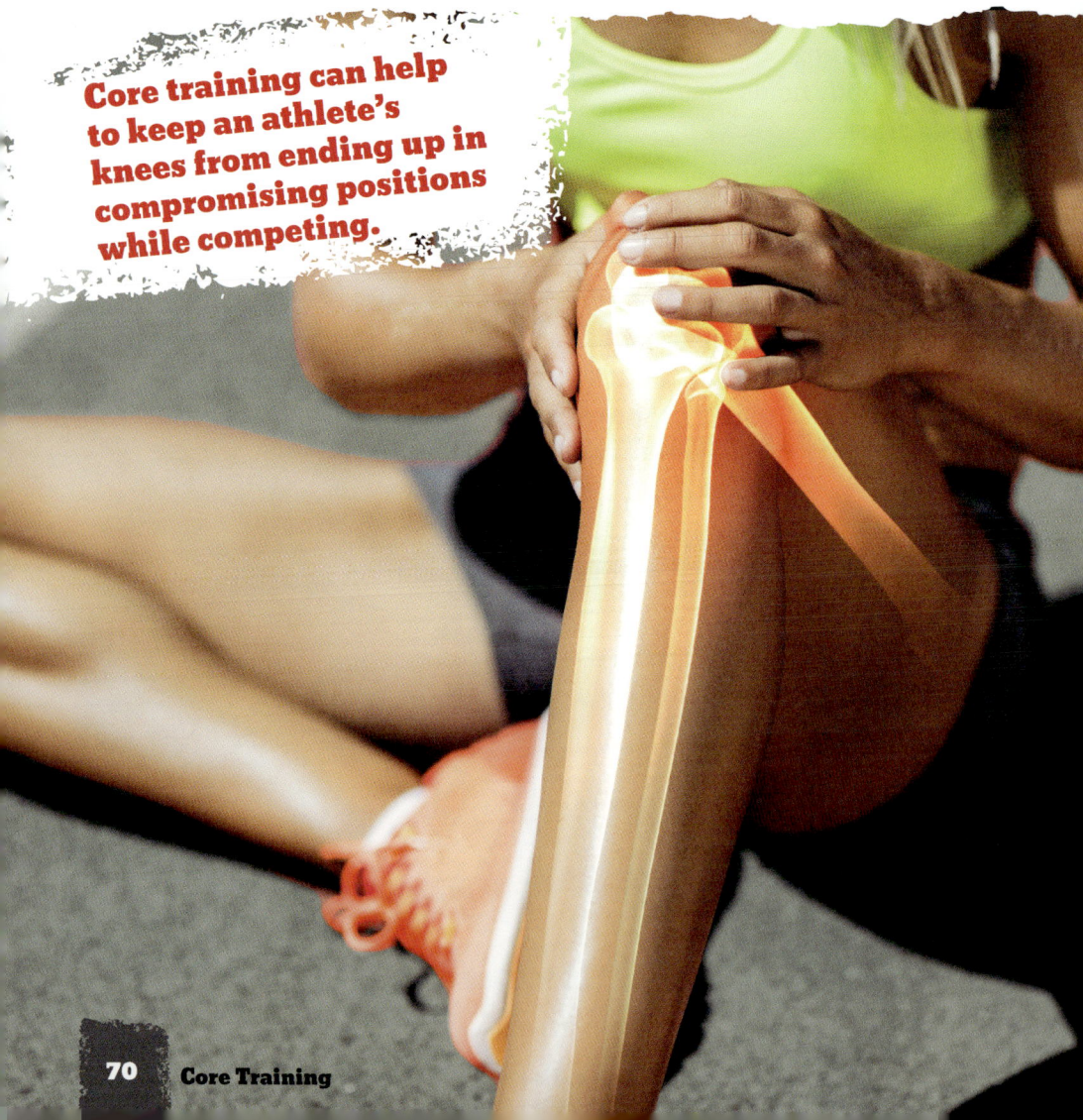

Core training can help to keep an athlete's knees from ending up in compromising positions while competing.

For example, a recent study showed that impaired core proprioception predicted knee injury risk in female athletes. Larger degrees of error in active repositioning correlated with knee ligament and meniscus injuries in particular. When another study looked at anterior cruciate ligament (ACL) rehabilitation, the previously injured group exhibited greater errors in trunk stability and control than healthy controls. These studies highlight the role of core stability in controlling the lumbopelvic–hip complex to limit unsafe displacement. Core training to prevent knee injury, therefore, requires teaching the neuromuscular system to generate and maintain stiffness through mobility.

As the knee is a lower-body joint, special attention should be paid to the load transfer muscles—in particular, the glutes, iliopsoas, and rectus abdominis. These muscles attach to the spine and the hip, and lack of good stability here can lead to injury further down the kinetic chain. To decrease injury risk, research from Kibler et al. suggests testing and training stability across various

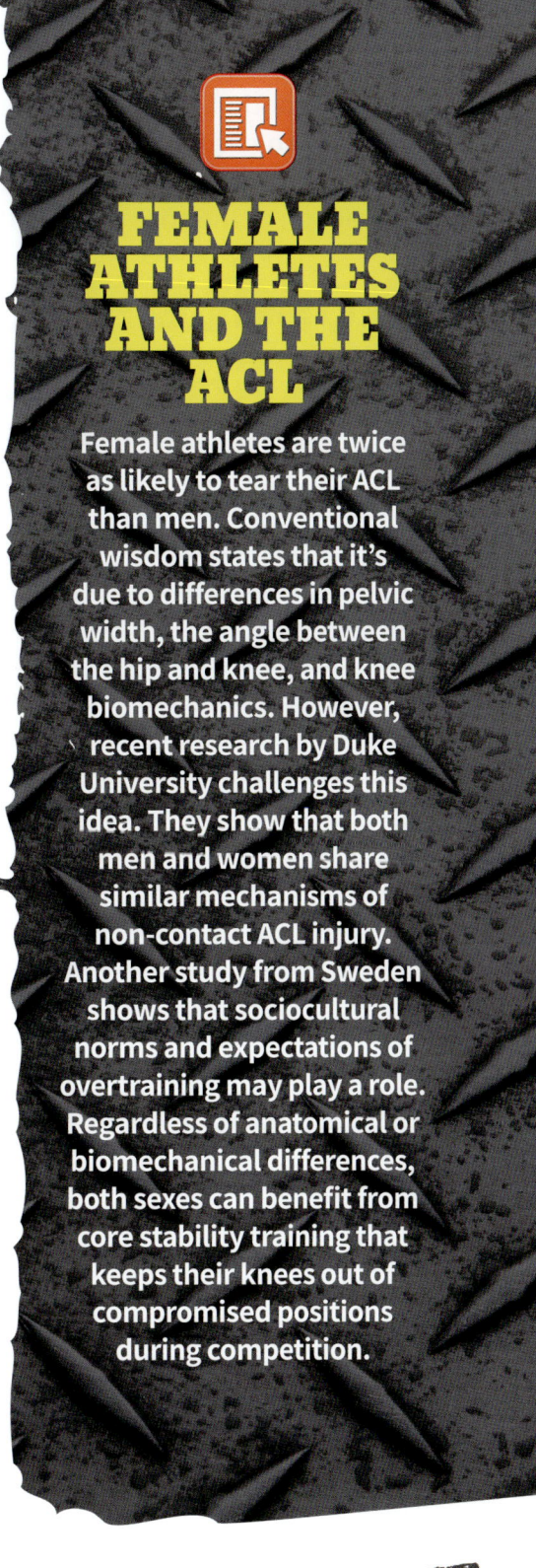

FEMALE ATHLETES AND THE ACL

Female athletes are twice as likely to tear their ACL than men. Conventional wisdom states that it's due to differences in pelvic width, the angle between the hip and knee, and knee biomechanics. However, recent research by Duke University challenges this idea. They show that both men and women share similar mechanisms of non-contact ACL injury. Another study from Sweden shows that sociocultural norms and expectations of overtraining may play a role. Regardless of anatomical or biomechanical differences, both sexes can benefit from core stability training that keeps their knees out of compromised positions during competition.

planes of motion. Examples include single-leg balancing, squatting, and deviating across three planes. Aim to minimize the use of your arms for balance, and reduce trunk and knee motion through contraction of the core musculature.

MUSCLE STRAINS OR TEARS (PELVIC ALIGNMENT)

It's common for muscles to strain or tear due to repetitive trauma. According to research, a lack of core strength and postural control has been shown to increase the risk of overuse injuries. Specifically, a decrease in side-to-side postural control, increased hip extension and strength, and muscular endurance contribute to injury prevention. Therefore, a comprehensive strength-training program includes exercises that challenge dynamic postural stability and isometric endurance. Such exercises include:

> Single-leg hip extension holds
> Planks with a shoulder tap
> Side planks
> Glute bridge marches
> Dead bugs
> Abdominal bracing

SHOULDER INJURIES

Due to anatomy, ligaments form the major attachments at the shoulder joint, with the muscles of the rotator cuff stabilizing the shoulder. As such, it naturally leans toward mobility and away from stability. However, with repetitive use, larger muscles will tighten up in an effort to protect the inner joint against degeneration. To avoid injury, mobility needs to be retained while maximizing rotator cuff and core stability. In a healthy shoulder, the rotator cuff locks things into place while big prime movers such as the lats, pecs, and deltoids control activity. Unfortunately, overuse leads to weak stabilizing muscles, poor positioning, and eventually undue strain.

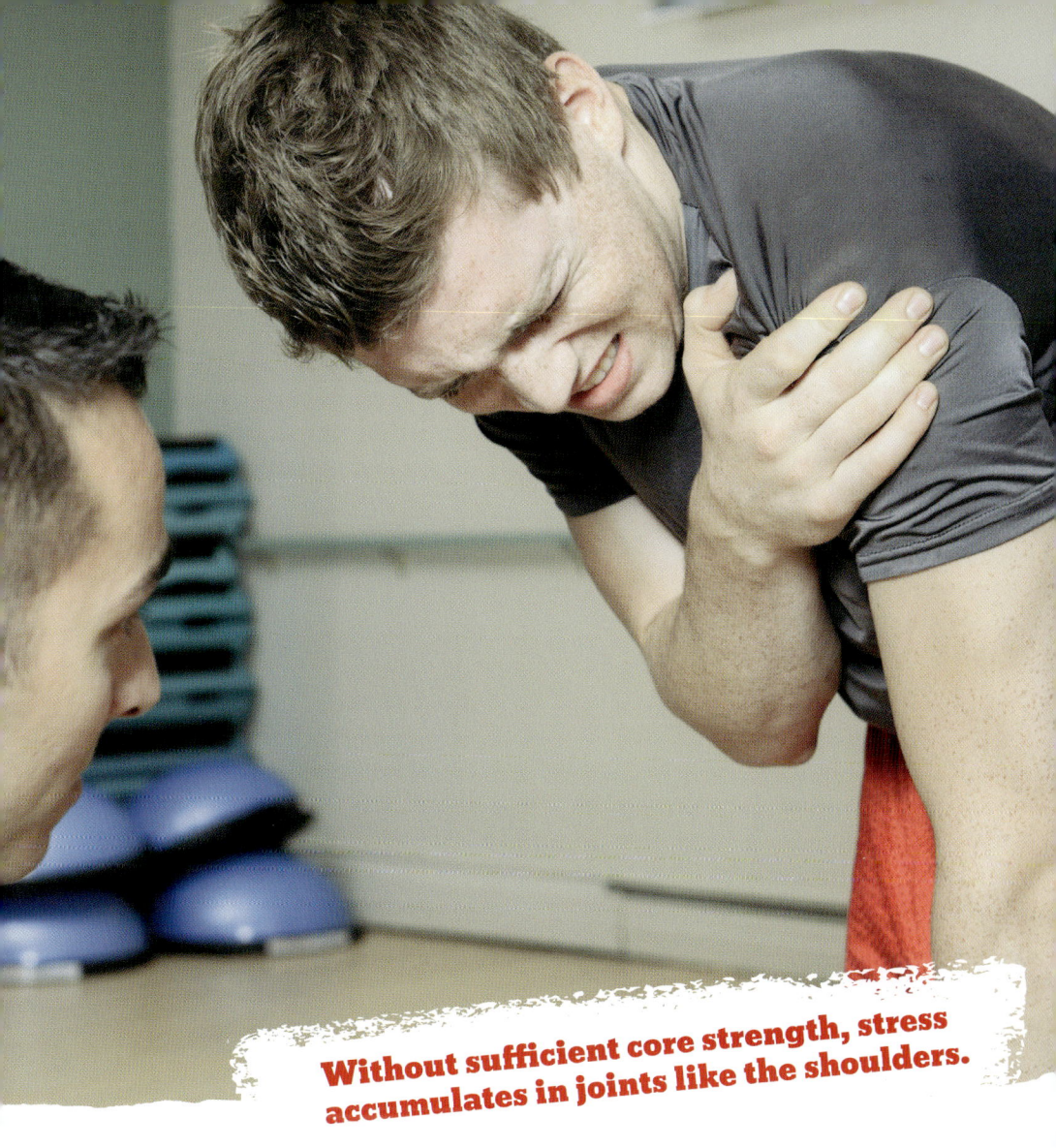

Without sufficient core strength, stress accumulates in joints like the shoulders.

Lifting weights, running, and throwing all require power transfer through the core into the joints. Without adequate core strength, stress accumulates at the shoulder during arm activity. To fully correct this imbalance, you need to train the core. Maximizing biomechanical efficiency will avoid overstressing the shoulder. Core strengthening exercises to improve shoulder health include Pallof pressing, scapular push-ups, and upside-down kettlebell carries.

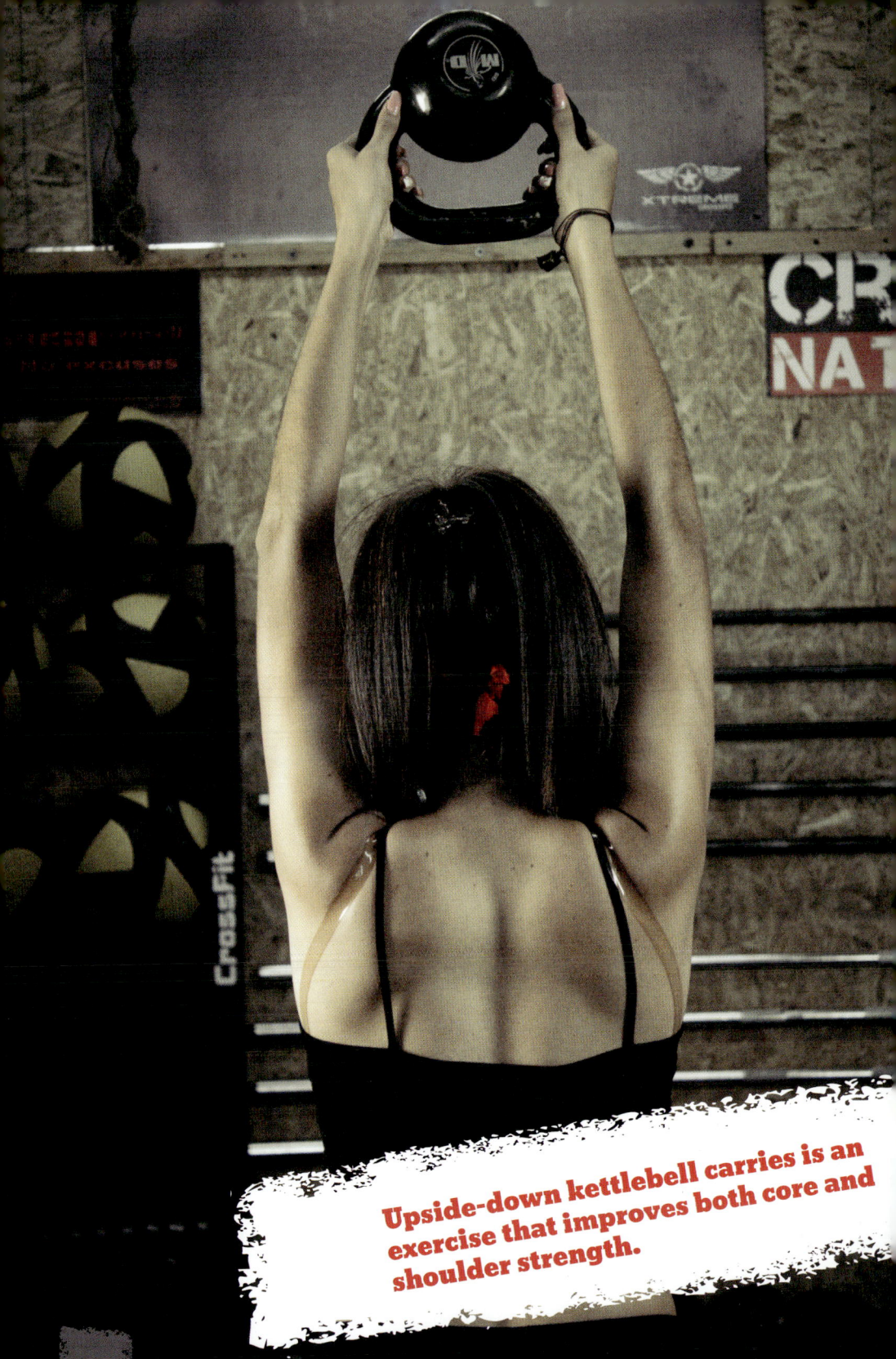

Upside-down kettlebell carries is an exercise that improves both core and shoulder strength.

Learn how to properly execute a basic upside-down kettlebell carry.

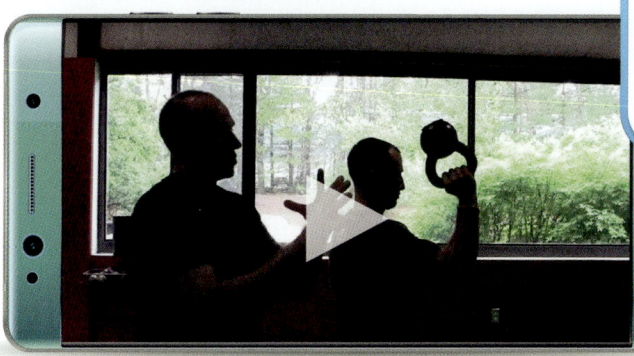

TEXT-DEPENDENT QUESTIONS

1. What's the difference between specific and non-specific lower back pain? Identify at least two contributors to each.

2. How can core training prevent knee injury? Identify two exercises to include in an injury prevention program.

3. How can biomechanical efficiency and postural control prevent both shoulder and overuse injuries?

RESEARCH PROJECT

Unfortunately, injuries happen sometimes despite our best efforts. Especially in high-level sports, injury risk is a part of the job. Research the most common injuries in both the Summer and Winter Olympics and choose one to expand upon. How would you train the core to (a) lessen injury risk and (b) rehabilitate an athlete from this injury?

WORDS TO UNDERSTAND

abdominal bracing—contraction of the abdominal muscles to create enough stiffness to prevent folding under load

anterior chain—a collection of muscles that work in tandem to control the front half of the body, such as the pectoralis major, quadriceps, and iliopsoas

posterior chain—a collection of muscles that work in tandem to control the back half of the body, such as glutes, hamstrings, and latissimus dorsi

spinal compression—a condition that puts pressure on your spinal cord and can cause numbness, tingling, pain, or weakness

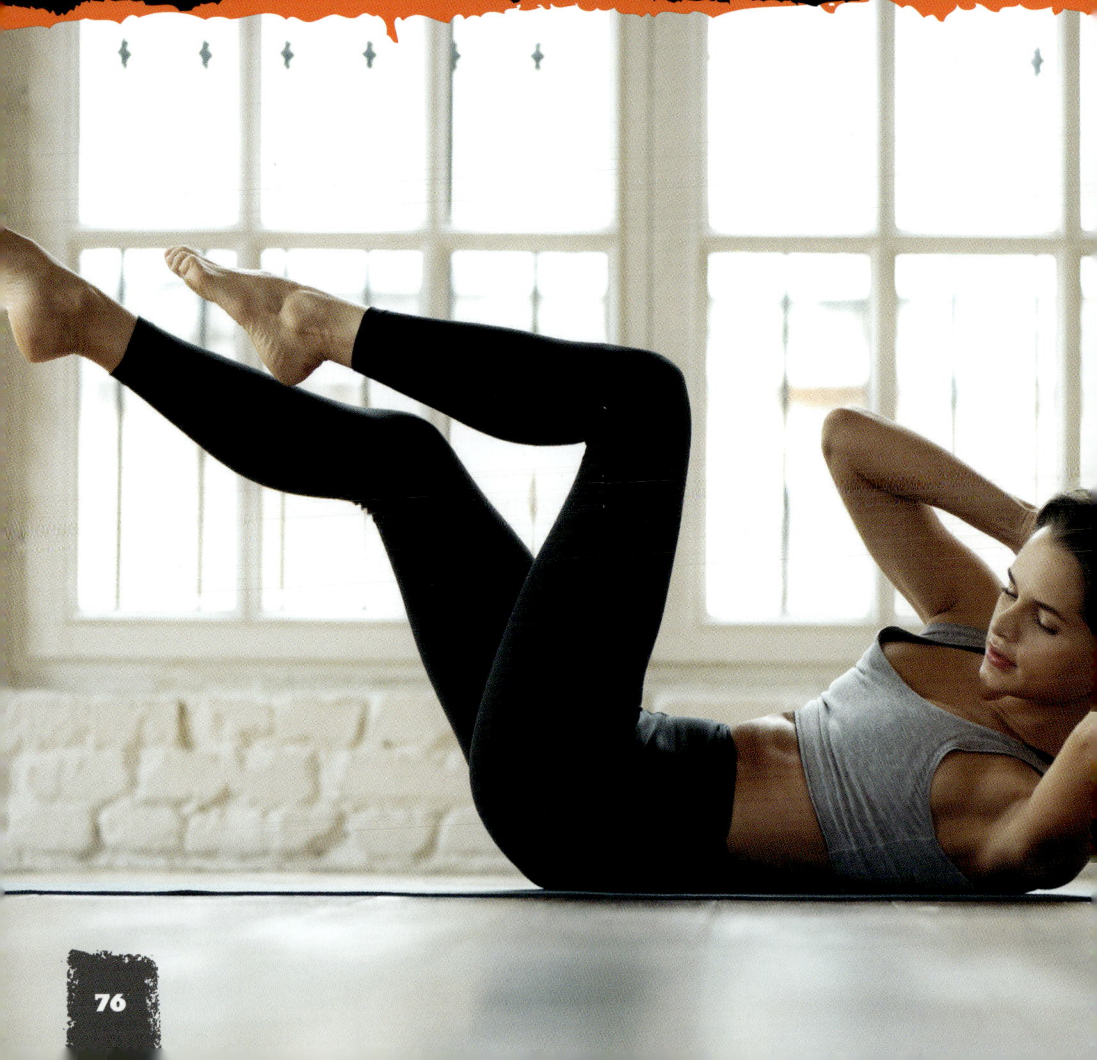

3. Brace your abdominals and punch straight away from your body. The band/cable should be pulling you back toward the anchor—don't let it. Resist the rotation and keep your arms extended straight in front of you.

4. Pause in extension and return to the start position. Complete for the prescribed amount of reps and repeat on the other side.

TEXT-DEPENDENT QUESTIONS

1. What is spinal compression and why do we want to avoid too much of it when training the core?

2. When would you use a lunge with rotation over the Pallof press and vice versa? Provide details behind your reasoning.

3. What muscles are primarily worked in a dead bug? A bird dog? Include applications for both in daily life.

RESEARCH PROJECT

Visit the ACE Exercise Library found under Internet Resources at the end of this book. Choose 3–5 core training exercises that are NOT mentioned earlier. Discuss the muscles worked and whether it trains local control, global stability, functional movement, or a combination. Then, pair those exercises with 3–5 exercises from this chapter to form a comprehensive, balanced core training program.

SERIES GLOSSARY OF KEY TERMS

Cardiorespiratory – of or relating to the heart and the respiratory system.

Circuit training – a workout technique involving a series of exercises performed in rotation with minimal rest, often using different pieces of apparatus.

Fatigue – weariness or exhaustion from labor, exertion, or stress.

HDL cholesterol – also known as good cholesterol. A lipoprotein of blood plasma that is composed of a high proportion of protein with little triglyceride and cholesterol and that is correlated with reduced risk of atherosclerosis.

Hormone – a product of living cells that circulates in body fluids (such as blood) and produces a specific and often stimulatory effect on the activity of cells, usually remote from its point of origin.

Lactic acid – a normally present hygroscopic organic acid ($C_3H_6O_3$), especially in muscle tissue, that is a by-product of anaerobic glycolysis, produced in carbohydrate matter usually by bacterial fermentation, and used especially in food and medicine and in industry.

LDL cholesterol – also known as bad cholesterol. A lipoprotein of blood plasma that is composed of a moderate proportion of protein with little triglyceride and a high proportion of cholesterol and that is associated with increased probability of developing atherosclerosis.

Metabolism – the chemical changes in living cells by which energy is provided for vital processes and activities, and new material is assimilated.

Micronutrients – a chemical element or substance (such as calcium or vitamin C) that is essential in minute amounts to the growth and health of a living organism.

Modification – the making of a limited change in something, such as an exercise, that makes the exercise easier.

Physiology – a branch of biology that deals with the functions and activities of life or of living matter (such as organs, tissues, or cells) and of the physical and chemical phenomena involved.

Resistance – of, relating to, or being an exercise involving pushing or pulling against the source of an opposing force (such as a weight) to increase strength.

Tempo – rate of motion or activity.

FURTHER READING

Joyce, D., and D. Lewindon. *Sports Injury Prevention and Rehabilitation Integrating Medicine and Science for Performance Solutions.* London: Routledge, 2016.

Liebman, H. *Anatomy of Core Stability.* Richmond, Ontario: Firefly Books, 2013.

Martin, Margaret. *Strengthen Your Core.* Kamajojo Press, 2013.

Moore, Rob. *100 Planks: The Plank Encyclopedia for Back Health, Bodyweight Training, and Ultimate Core Strength.* 2019.

National Strength & Conditioning Association (NSCA). *Developing the Core.* Champaign: Human Kinetics Publishers, 2013.

INTERNET RESOURCES

https://breakingmuscle.com/learn/how-are-we-still-getting-it-wrong-abdominal-hollowing-vs-bracing

Breaking Muscle is an online platform for information on exercise, fitness, and nutrition. In this article, they discuss the importance of abdominal bracing in creating intra-abdominal pressure and stability.

https://www.acefitness.org/education-and-resources/lifestyle/exercise-library

American Council on Exercise (ACE) is a reputable fitness accreditation organization that provides a library of exercise instruction.

https://www.backfitpro.com

BackFitPro is the website for Dr. Stuart McGill, Dr. Edward Cambridge, and Joel Proskewitz—three industry-leading experts on core stability and back pain.

https://www.functionalmovement.com

Functional Movement Systems is the home of the original Functional Movement Screen and all related resources.

https://simplifaster.com/articles/core-training-programs-athletic-performance

SimpliFaster is a company dedicated to speed and athletic performance. Their blog regularly features sports performance articles, such as this one on core training for athletes.

INDEX

A

Abdominal bracing, 77–78
Abs (abdominals), 14, 15, 21, 78
Afferent neurons, 48
Anterior cruciate ligament (ACL) rehabilitation, 71
Anti-movement exercises, 59
Anticipatory postural adjustments, 47–48
Assessments (static/dynamic), of core strength, 30–36
Athletic performance, 11–13
Athleticism, 53

B

Backward medicine ball toss test, 35
Balance, core role in, 14–15
Bench press, 12
Bird dogs, 78–80
BMX racing, 61
Bodyweight, 11
Bracing
 abdominal, 77–78
 positional, 54
Breathing, diaphragmatic, 44–45, 77

C

Central nervous system (CNS), 47
Comprehensive strength-training program, 72
Contact sports, 59–61
Cook, Gray, 38, 43
Core
 anatomy and biomechanics, 17–27
 in balance, 14–15
 description of, 7
 difficulties to defining, 8
 local and global systems of, 8
 muscles, 14, 17, 50
 role in stabilizing against movement, 45–51
 workouts, 11, 15
Core endurance, 57
Core stability
 defined, 43
 improving, 11–13
 measuring, 36–41
 science of, 43–51

single-leg balance assessment, 39–41
training, 51
unilateral hip bridge assessment, 36, 38
Core strength
 dynamic assessments of, 32–36
 exercises, 73–74
 improving, 11–13
 measuring, 29–36
 static assessments of, 29–31
Core training
 athletic performance, 11–13
 for athleticism, 53–63
 benefits of, 11–15
 contact sports, 59–61
 endurance sports, 57–59
 exercises, 77–91
 functional movements, 85–91
 global stabilization exercises, 78–84
 improved balance, 14–15
 injury prevention, 13–14, 65–75
 local control exercises, 77–78
 for non-contact team sports, 55–57
 physique development, 15
 power sports, 59
 trick-based sports, 61–63
 workouts, 11
 See also Sport-specific core training
Cycling output and core stability, 14

D

Dead bug exercise, 80–81
Deadlifts, 13
Deceleration, 55
Diaphragm, 19–20
Diaphragmatic breathing, 44–45, 77
Duke University, 71
Dynamic assessments of core strength
 backward medicine ball toss test, 35
 forward medicine ball toss test, 32, 35
 isokinetic exercises, 32

medicine ball tests, 32
rotational medicine ball toss test, 36
Dynamic functional movements, examples for, 66
Dynamometers, 32

E

Efferent neurons, 48
Endurance sports, 57–59
Erector spinae, 23–24
External obliques, 22

F

Fascia, 21
Fatigue, 63
Feed-forward core contractions, 47, 48
Feed-forward reactions, 17, 19
Female athletes, knee injury risk in, 71
Forward medicine ball toss test, 32, 35
Front plank exercise, 81–82
Functional Movement Screen, 38, 65
Functional movements
 examples for, 66
 lunges with rotation, 87–89
 McGill Curl-up, 86–87
 Pallof press, 89–91
 weighted carries, 85–86

G

Global muscles, 8
Global stabilization
 exercises, 66, 68
 bird dogs, 78–80
 dead bugs, 80–81
 examples for, 65
 front plank, 81–82
 glute bridge, 83–84
 side plank, 82–83
 See also Core stability
Glute bridges, 83–84
Glutes, 24, 27, 83–84
Gluteus maximus, 27
 in lower body movements, 69
Gluteus medius, 27
Gluteus minimus, 27
Gymnasts, 62–63

I

Iliacus, 23
Iliocostalis, 24
Iliopsoas, 23
Injury prevention, 13–14, 65–75
    knee, 70–72
    lower back pain, 66–69
    pelvic alignment, 72
    shoulder, 72
"Inner core", 47
Internal obliques, 21–22
International Journal of Sports Physical Therapy, 65
Inverted kettlebell carry, 85
Isokinetic exercises, 32
Isometric dynamometers, 32

J

Journal of Strength and Conditioning, 61

K

Kicking action, 18
Knee injuries, 70–72

L

Lateral flexion, 22
Lateral musculature test, 30–31
Load transfer muscles, 51
Local and global postural control, 53–54
Local and global systems of core, 8
Local control exercises
    abdominal bracing, 77–78
    diaphragmatic breathing, 77
Longissimus, 24
Lower back pain, 66–69
    examples to preventing, 69
Lunges with rotation, 87–89

M

McGill, Stuart, 29, 86
McGill Curl-up, 86–87
Medicine ball tests, 32
Motor performance, 53
Movement (book by Cook), 38
Movement economy, improving, 58–59
Multifidus, 19
Muscle strains or tears, 72

N

Neuromuscular control exercises, examples for, 65
Non-contact team sports, core training for, 55–57
Non-specific lower back pain, 67

O

Obliques, 15, 36
    external and internal, 21–22
Olympic lifts, 13
One-sided carries, 85
"Outer core", 48

P

Pallof press, 73, 89–91
Panjabi, M. M., 45
Pelvic alignment, 72
Pelvic floor muscles, 19
Pelvic tilt, 23, 32, 33
Physique development, 15
Plank exercises, 69
Positional bracing, 54
Postural alignment, in standing, 32
Power sports, 59
Power transfer, core training for, 54–55
Psoas major, 23

Q

Quadratus lumborum (QL), 24, 26
Quarterbacks, 54

R

Reactionary postural adjustments, 48–49
Rectus abdominis, 8, 9, 14, 15, 21
Rotation
    lunges with, 87–89
    of upper body, 22, 89
Rotational medicine ball toss test, 36, 37
Rotator cuff, 72

S

Scapular push-ups, 73
Sensory receptors, 48
Shoulder injuries, 72
Side plank exercise, 82–83
Singer, Bob, 53
Single-leg balance/squat test, 39–41, 55, 57
Sit-up test, 29
Soccer, 56
Specific lower back pain, 67
Spinal compression, 87
Spinal extension, 24
Spinal flexion, 21
Spinalis, 24
Sport-specific core training
    deceleration, 55
    local and global postural control, 53–54
    positional bracing, 54
    power transfer, 54–55
Sports Medicine journal, 12
Squat position, 41
Squats, 13, 43
Stability
    defined, 43
    and postural control, 49
Stabilization exercises, 66
    bird dogs, 78–80
    dead bugs, 80–81
    examples for, 65
    front plank, 81–82
    glute bridge, 83–84
    side plank, 82–83
    See also Core stability
Standing postural alignment, 32
Static assessments of core strength
    lateral musculature test, 30–31
    trunk extensor test (TFT), 30
    trunk flexor test (TFT), 30
Static tissue, 45
Stress, 73
Supercross BMX, 61

T

Test-retest reliability, 32
Thoracolumbar fascia, 21
Transverse abdominis (TVA), 8, 11, 17–19, 65
Trick-based sports, 61–63
Trunk extensor test (TET), 30, 68
Trunk flexor test (TFT), 30

U

Unilateral hip bridge endurance test, 36, 38, 39
University of Pittsburgh, 32
Upside-down kettlebell carries, 73, 74

W

Weighted carries, 85–86
Weightlifting, 10, 11
Workouts, 11, 15, 24

AUTHOR BIOGRAPHY

Kimber Rozier is a NSCA certified strength and conditioning specialist who holds dual Bachelor's degrees in Exercise and Sport Science and Spanish, as well as a professional athlete competing with the USA women's national rugby team. In 2013, she earned a bronze medal at the Rugby 7s Women's World Cup in Moscow and competed in the 2014 15s World Cup in Paris and 2017 World Cup in Ireland. As an entrepreneur, former Harvard coach, and decorated professional rugby player, she loves sharing her knowledge through coaching and writing. Certified by the NSCA and Precision Nutrition, she brings her wealth of experience to the page, sharpening the lens by which we see the world. She writes for multiple small health and wellness businesses, as well as large publications such as Men's Health, MyFitnessPal, and EliteFTS. She now owns her own business, Dare Performance, in which she promotes a healthy lifestyle through journalism.

PHOTO CREDITS

Shutterstock.com
Pg. 1: AVAVA, 3, 6, 37, 55: Jacob Lund, 9: Anatomy Insider, 12: Maksim Toome, 13: Jacek Chabraszewski, 14: iko, 18: Fotokostic, 20: sciencepics, 22: Prostock-studio, 23, 88: Maridav, 25, 33: Sebastian Kaulitzki, 26: Gang Liu, 28: sirtravelalot, 34: Alan Poulson Photography, 39: Aleksandr Kondratov, 40: Nadir Keklik, 52: UfaBizPhoto, 56: Photo Works, 66: Evannovostro, 68, 76: fizkes, 69: Syda Productions, 70: wavebreakmedia, 73: Lopolo, 7 Kjetil Kolbjornsrud, 81: Undrey, 84: Undray, 86: baranq, 90: oneinchpunch

Dreamstime.com
Pg. 10: Monkey Business Images, 6: Undrey, 42: Jeff Cleveland, 44: Vadim Zakharishchev, 46: Chrischrisw, 47: Sergey Novikov, 48: Rostislav Zatonskiy, 50: Martinmark, 60: Jbcalom, 62: Galina Barskaya, 64: motortion, 74: Mauricio Ledesma, 82: Ozimician

Flickr
Pg. 54: KA Sports Photos
Pg. 58: mluke123

EDUCATIONAL VIDEO LINKS

Chapter 1: http://x-qr.net/1Lx8
Chapter 2: http://x-qr.net/1KaN
Chapter 3: http://x-qr.net/1JMU, http://x-qr.net/1M4y, http://x-qr.net/1LB3
Chapter 4: http://x-qr.net/1Lgx
Chapter 5: http://x-qr.net/1L12
Chapter 6: http://x-qr.net/1LHA, http://x-qr.net/1K1F
Chapter 7: http://x-qr.net/1LV7

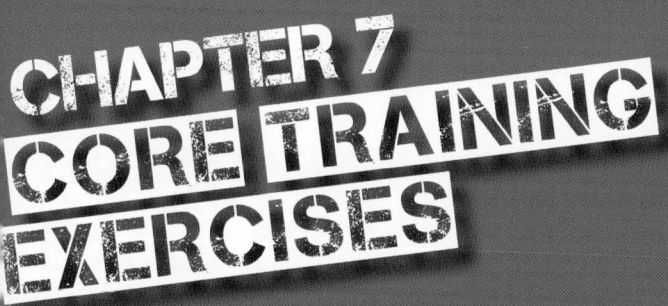

LOCAL CONTROL EXERCISES

Diaphragmatic Breathing

As mentioned in previous chapters, diaphragmatic breathing sets up the foundation for core stability. So how do you know if you're breathing well? The easiest way is to lie on your back, place your one hand over your stomach, one on your chest, and inhale. In diaphragmatic breathing, you'll feel your stomach rise with one hand while the other stays put. In contrast, breathing into your chest will cause the wrong hand to rise.

Once you've mastered diaphragmatic breathing, it's critical to maintain throughout all other bracing, stability, or functional exercises. Breathing is the one action that permeates all movements. Get it right, and you'll be on your way to total body performance.

Abdominal Bracing

Have you ever thought you were going to be hit in the stomach? Hopefully not, but your gut reaction would be to brace your abdomen. In contrast to hollowing, which focuses solely on contracting the transverse abdominis, **abdominal bracing** contracts the entire core as one. This ensures that we're training stiffness that transfers to real life. All sides of your core cylinder stiffen up to protect the spine, providing stability across all planes of movement.

 Learn about the importance of abdominal bracing in this video.

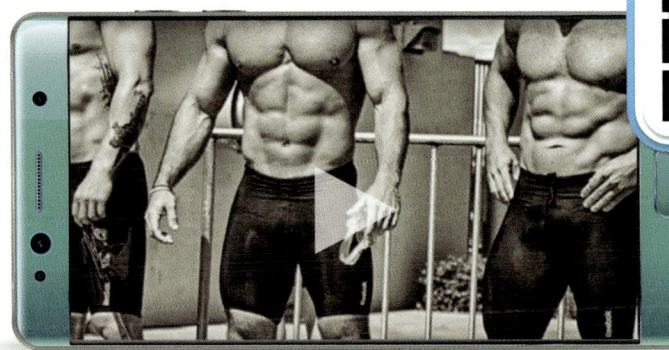

To correctly brace the abdomen, lie on your back with your shoulders relaxed, down, and back. Bend the knees to 90° with feet flat on the floor. Squeeze the glutes to set the pelvis in position, and then stiffen your abs as if you were about to get punched. Avoid exaggerating—this should be a gentle yet firm contraction. Make sure you're able to practice diaphragmatic breathing while maintaining this position. From there, practice bracing from sitting, kneeling, and then standing.

GLOBAL STABILIZATION EXERCISES

Bird Dogs

Start in the quadruped position on all fours on the floor. Make sure your shoulders are stacked above your wrists and knee underneath the hips. Your spine should begin in neutral and remain that way throughout. A good test to discover neutral is placing a PVC pipe on the back so that it touches the base of the head, the mid-back, and the hips.

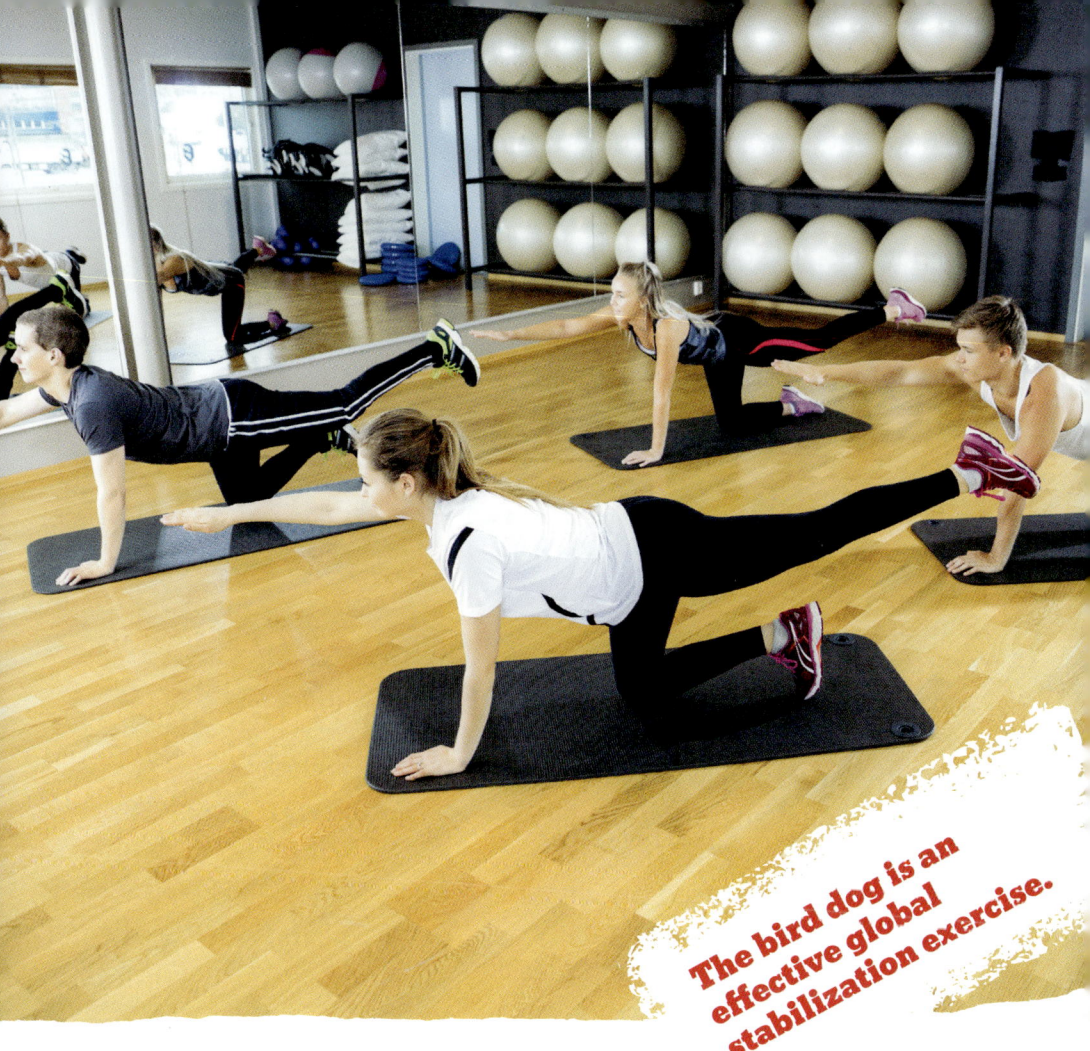

The bird dog is an effective global stabilization exercise.

To begin a bird dog, follow these steps:

1. Gradually extend your right leg behind you as if you were trying to plant your foot flat on the wall. At the same time, reach your left arm overhead in front of you. Avoid shrugging your shoulder to your ears as you do so.

2. Keep your hips and shoulders square with a neutral spine as you fully extend opposite sides. Pause briefly at the top, making sure you're not overarching the back.

3. Slowly return opposite arm and leg to the starting position until you're on all fours. Repeat the motion on the opposite side.

Once you get comfortable with one controlled movement per side, feel free to complete multiple reps before switching. Just make sure you don't succumb to fatigue or tilt away from neutral.

Dead Bugs

Similar to the bird dog, the dead bug exercise asks you to alternate arm and leg movement. However, you'll do so lying on your back. As you're facing the opposite direction, this movement challenges the stability of your **anterior chain**. The goal is to keep your core braced the whole time while fighting against gravity and the shifts in your center of mass.

To perform a dead bug, follow these steps:

1. Lie down on your back, bend the knees, and take a deep breath to relax. First set yourself with diaphragmatic breathing and bracing.
2. From there, lift the feet until your shins are parallel to the floor, knees over the hips. At the same time, lift both arms overhead, wrists stacked above your shoulders. From the outside, you should look like you're trying to crawl on the ceiling.

WHY BIRD DOGS AND DEAD BUGS?

Have you ever seen a pointer dog out on the hunt? Once its owner shoots down a bird, it's the dog's job to find the game and point it out to the hunter. As they don't have fingers, bird dogs point with their bodies, lifting one leg off the ground with the opposite leg back, extending as far as possible (hence the name of the exercise). Dead bugs often go belly-up, kicking their little legs in the air. At the start of the exercise, therefore, it's said you look like a dead bug. Despite the macabre analogy, these exercises are staples of helping to optimize functional human movement.

3. Initiate movement by slowly straightening and lowering your right leg and left arm. Keep the opposite limbs facing the ceiling. Continue lowering until your right leg and left arm are fully extended a few inches away from the floor. Avoid rib flare, pelvic tilt, or any arching of the back as you do so.
4. Reverse the movement to the start position and repeat on the other side. Continue until you've completed all required reps.

Front Plank

Holding a plank continues to be a display of core strength and endurance. It's one of the more difficult exercises to challenge stiffness over time. Rather than maintaining position through motion, a plank requires the core to fight against the pull of gravity.

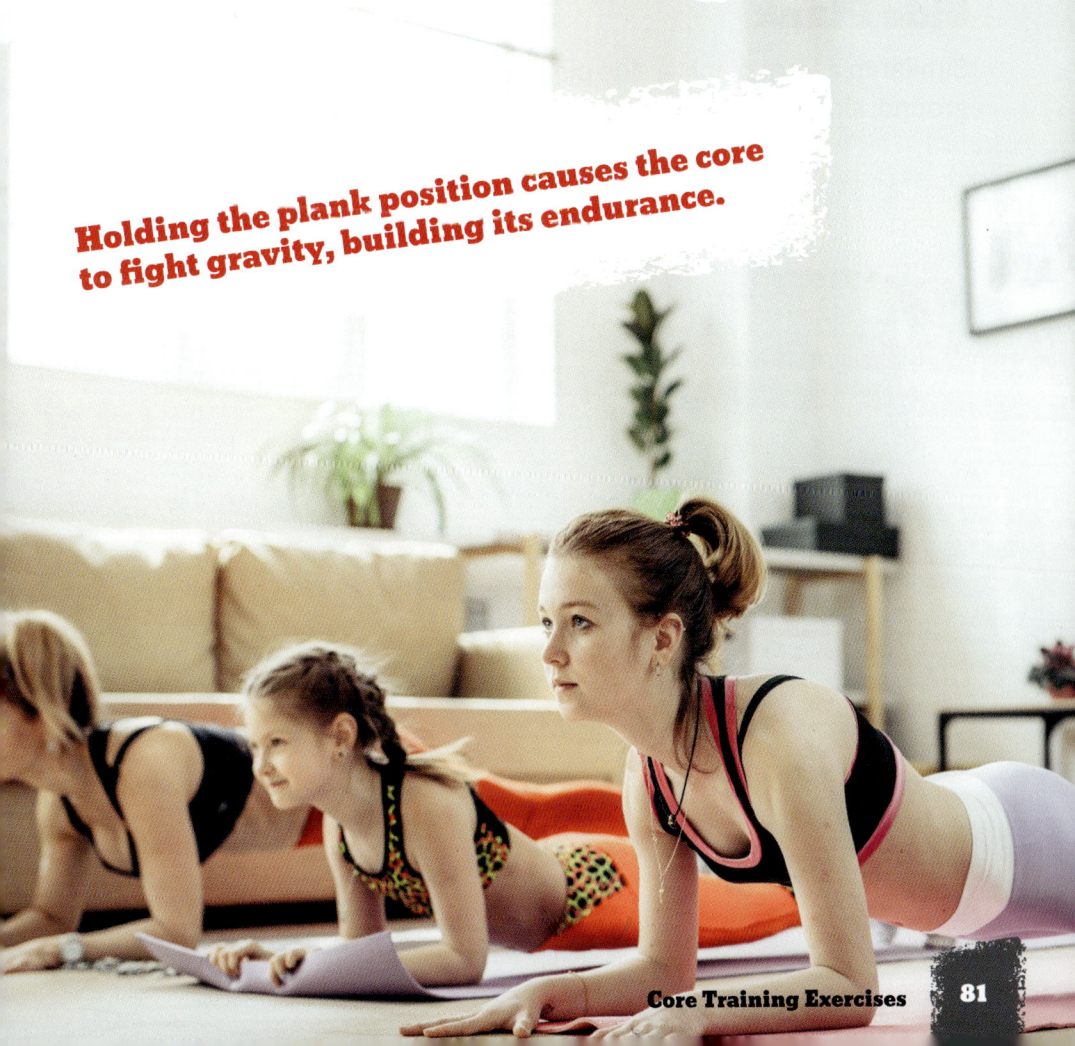

Holding the plank position causes the core to fight gravity, building its endurance.

With only two points of contact, it creates a long lever, supported only by your abs. A front plank works your transverse abdominis, rectus abdominis, glutes, obliques, and other muscles.

To complete a front plank, follow these steps:

1. Set up in a push-up position, with feet hip-width apart and wrists underneath the shoulders. Make sure your body forms a straight line between the heels and the head. Then, drop to your elbows with forearms resting on the ground.
2. Maintain a neutral spine by squeezing the glutes, tucking the pelvis, bracing the abdominals, and pulling your shoulder blades down.
3. Stay active in this position as long as possible. One rep is complete when time runs out, or you can no longer maintain a neutral spine.

Side Plank

Similar to a front plank, a side plank aims to lift the body off of the ground, similar to a bridge. However, a side plank is performed with one

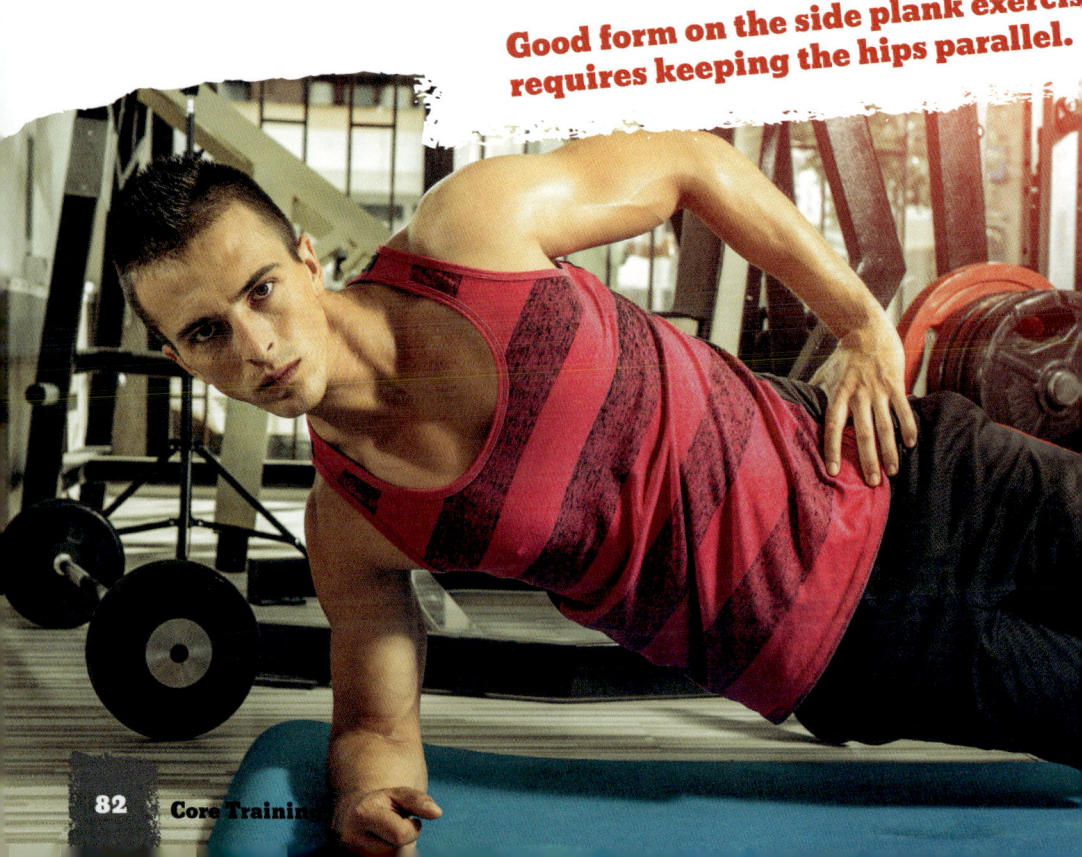

Good form on the side plank exercise requires keeping the hips parallel.

elbow on the floor and feet stacked. If that's uncomfortable, place one foot slightly in front of the other.

To perform a side plank,

1. Lay on the floor on your side. Elevate yourself up on one elbow, lifting the hips into the air with feet planted. Make sure your shoulders stay stacked above the elbow without any deviation. Hips and shoulders should remain perpendicular to the ground and parallel to each other.
2. Continue to create space under the hips by activating the obliques and lateral glutes.
3. Hold this position until the hips drop below parallel or time expires.

Glute Bridge

As a fantastic core exercise, the glute bridge challenges the endurance of your **posterior chain**. If performed correctly, it'll engage your glutes, multifidus, quadratus lumborum, erectors, and obliques.

To execute a glute bridge, follow these steps:

1. Lie on your back and bend your knees at 90° with feet flat on the floor. Completely brace the core before moving, making sure you can breathe comfortably through the diaphragm. Then, squeeze the glutes and press through your heels.
2. Think about lifting one vertebra off the floor at a time. This helps to keep your core pillar stacked. When your hips reach full extension, stop and fully squeeze your glutes. Make sure not to arch the back to avoid hyperextension. Additionally, avoid tilting the hips toward either side.
3. Slowly lower the hips back to the floor to complete one rep. Complete for the prescribed number of reps or hold at the top for an endurance challenge.

To add even more of a challenge, march your heels at the top. Keeping one heel planted on the floor, lift the other foot, bringing

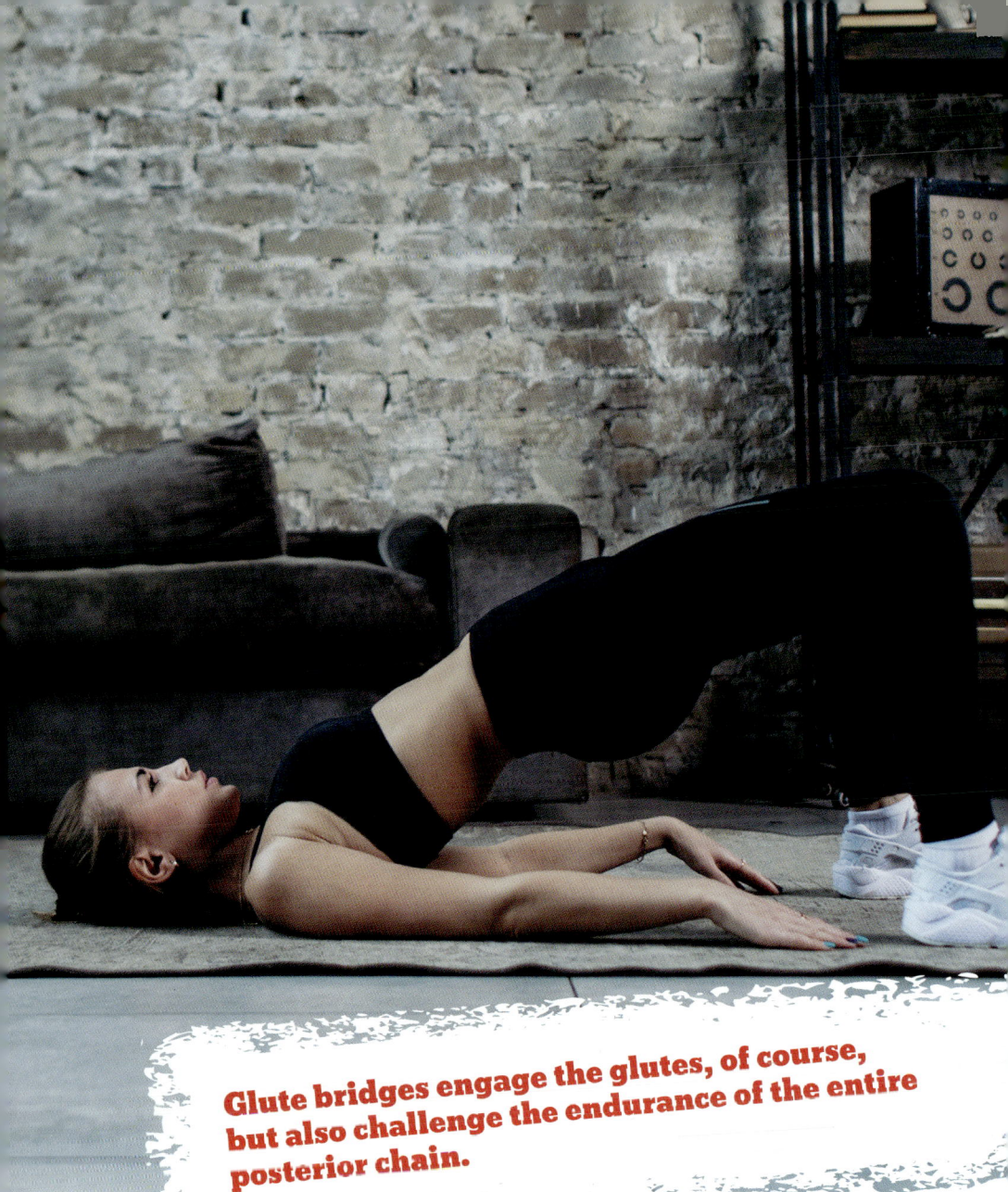

Glute bridges engage the glutes, of course, but also challenge the endurance of the entire posterior chain.

your knee toward your chest. Your body will try to tilt in response to the instability. Keep squeezing your planted glute to stay in extension and tighten your core to resist rotation. Slowly lower your heel back to the floor and repeat on the other side. Remember, only your legs should be moving. The core should remain stable throughout.

FUNCTIONAL MOVEMENTS

Weighted Carries

Weighted carries help develop a solid core brace to protect the spine under load. Sports, certain careers, and everyday life demand safely manipulating external loads. Weighted carries place the upper back under tension while walking, challenging you to maintain balance and stability. One-sided carries test especially anti-lateral flexion and rotation. The added weight naturally pulls your core to tilt away from center and your muscles fight hard to stay neutral.

To properly execute a weighted carry, follow these steps:

1. Grab two weights of a moderate-to-heavy load and hold them tight to your side. With shoulders down and back, brace your core to create tension before movement.
2. Walk forward for the prescribed distance, maintaining a tall posture and neutral spine, and carefully set the weights down at the end.

Variations on the weighted carry include:

1. **One-sided carries**: Grab a heavy dumbbell or kettlebell and carry it on one side only. Fight to keep your shoulders and hips parallel as the weight tries to pull you down. You can also increase the weight or distance to ramp up the intensity.
2. **Inverted kettlebell carry**: Grab a lighter kettlebell and hold it upside down in one arm with a bent elbow. Keeping the shoulder blade packed and elbow out in front, fight to keep the kettlebell in position while walking forward. You should feel the instability in your shoulder as well as in your core.

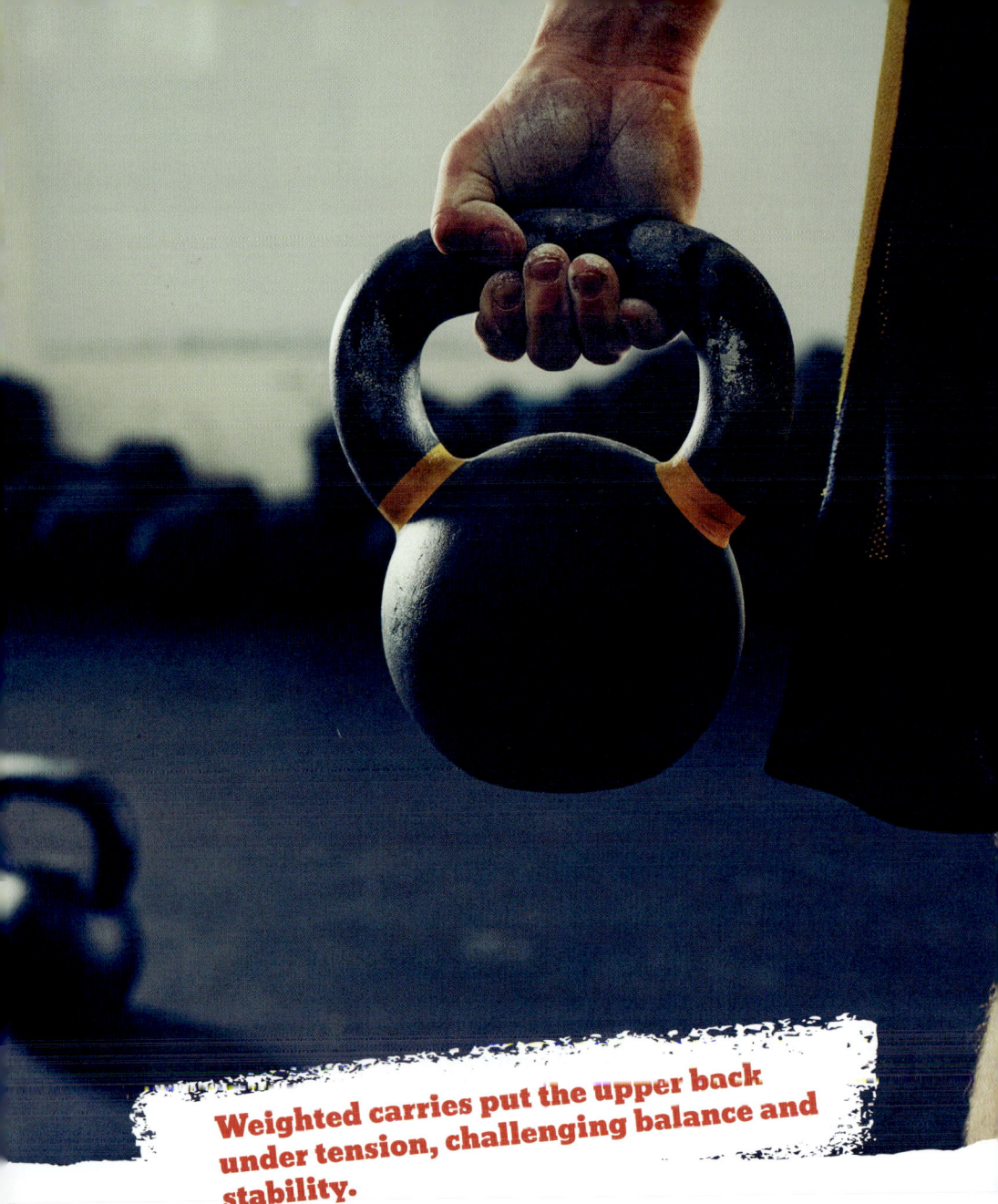

Weighted carries put the upper back under tension, challenging balance and stability.

McGill Curl-Up

Stuart McGill, Ph.D., is one of the leading experts on core stability. Throughout his research, he invented a safer, more effective version of the sit-up—the McGill Curl-up. It's been shown to develop greater core stiffness while reducing hip flexor activity and **spinal compression**. This makes it an ideal option for those with lower back pain, and it helps work the entire anterior cylinder as a unit.

To perform the McGill Curl-up, follow these steps:

1. Lie on your back with one leg bent to 90°, the other completely straight. Before movement, place both hands underneath the arch of your lower back.
2. Brace your core, and slowly elevate your head and shoulder blades off of the floor. Once your shoulder blades clear the ground, pause and hold.
3. Notice that you're not sitting all the way up to the knees. Rather, it's a small contraction of the abdominals to elevate your shoulders and head. Take care to relax the neck as much as possible, focusing on the tension in your abs.
4. Hold for 5–10 seconds per rep and then slowly return to the ground. Complete the prescribed reps and then switch sides.

Lunge with Rotation

Any sport that warrants upright, dynamic movement should train lunges with rotation. The lunge naturally puts you on an unstable base, with each leg fighting to counterbalance the other. This split stance mimics the demands of running, walking, kicking, or any other variation of upright motion. To protect your pelvis and lower back, the upper and lower extremities should operate independently. Being able to plant your feet firmly during a pitch, for example, increases maximum throwing velocity. Even non-athletes can benefit from greater body control, and this is one of the more functional ways to train that.

Lunges with a rotation should be executed with a light to moderate weight. It's not an upper body strength exercise. You shouldn't be struggling to hold the dumbbell or medicine ball in your hands beforehand. Rather, aim for something in the 10–25 pound range, depending on body weight, size, and existing core strength.

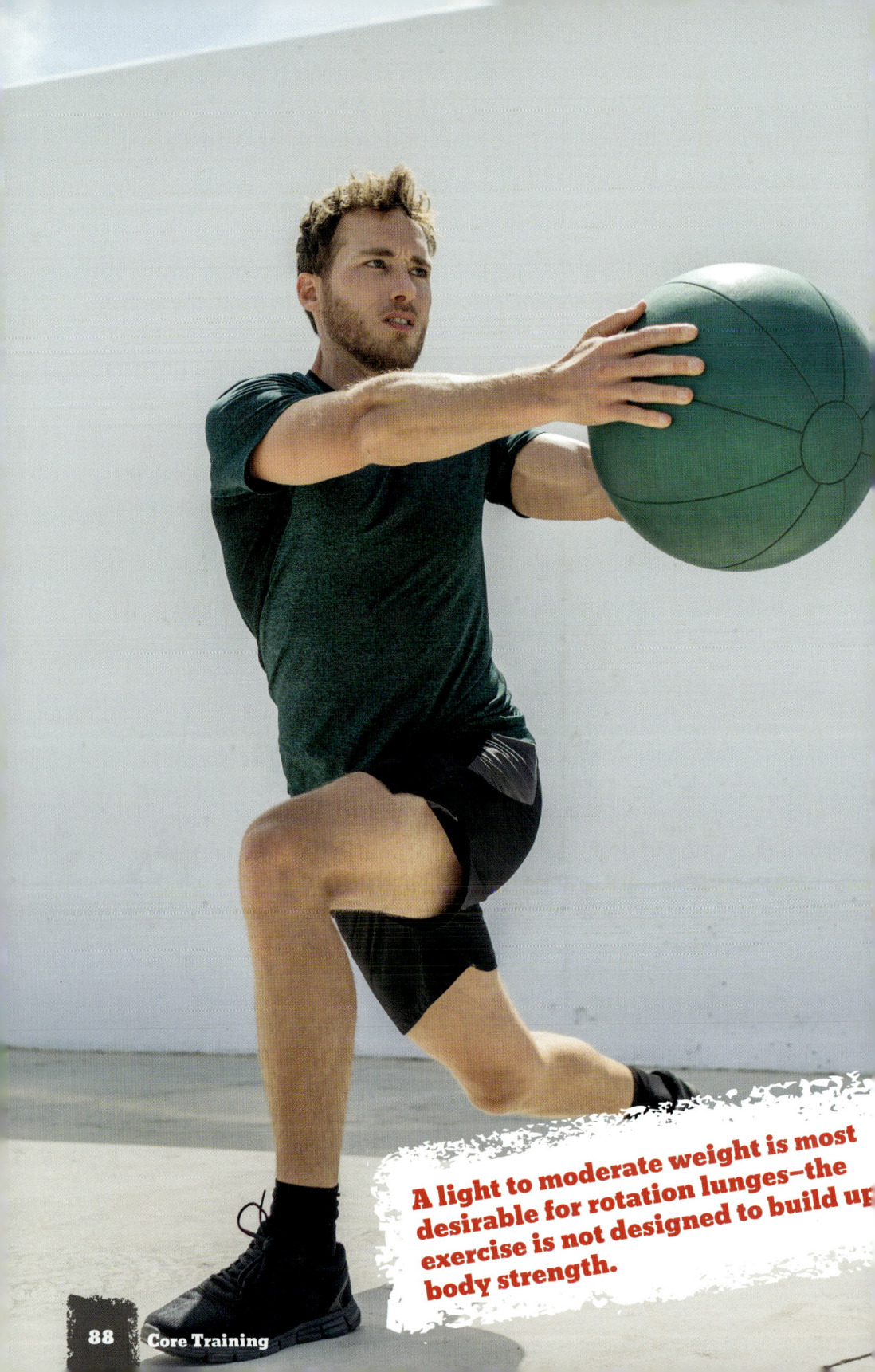

A light to moderate weight is most desirable for rotation lunges—the exercise is not designed to build up body strength.

To perform a lunge with rotation, follow these steps:

1. Begin standing tall, holding a weight in both hands, feet hip-width apart.
2. Extend your arms straight out in front of you so that they're parallel with the ground.
3. Step one foot forward into a lunge, planting the front foot flat on the floor, and bending that knee to 90°.
4. Keeping the arms straight, rotate your torso across the front leg. You should now be facing the same side as the leg you stepped with. Pause for a second or two.
5. Carefully rotate back to center, press through your feet, and return to standing. Repeat on the other side, and continue for the prescribed amount of reps.

Pallof Press

The Pallof press is a great way to train midline stability while standing upright. In this exercise, you're fighting against rotation through varying levels of resistance. It works the rectus abdominis, obliques, and total torso anti-rotation. Moving your arms trains the core to stay locked in despite external motion disturbances. Functionally, this type of neuromuscular control transfers to lifting, sports, and everyday life. Controlling excessive upper body rotation in a sprint, for example, improves running economy. A tight, solid foundation increases pressing strength in the gym. And resisting rotation can protect the spine when moving groceries, lifting suitcases, playing with the dog, or rearranging furniture.

To perform a Pallof press, follow these steps:

1. Secure a resistance band around an anchor at belly button height or adjust a cable machine to the same level. Grab the end of the band/cable and stand at a 90° angle to its anchor.
2. With feet hip-width apart, glutes engaged, and knees relaxed, bring the band/cable to your belly button with both hands.

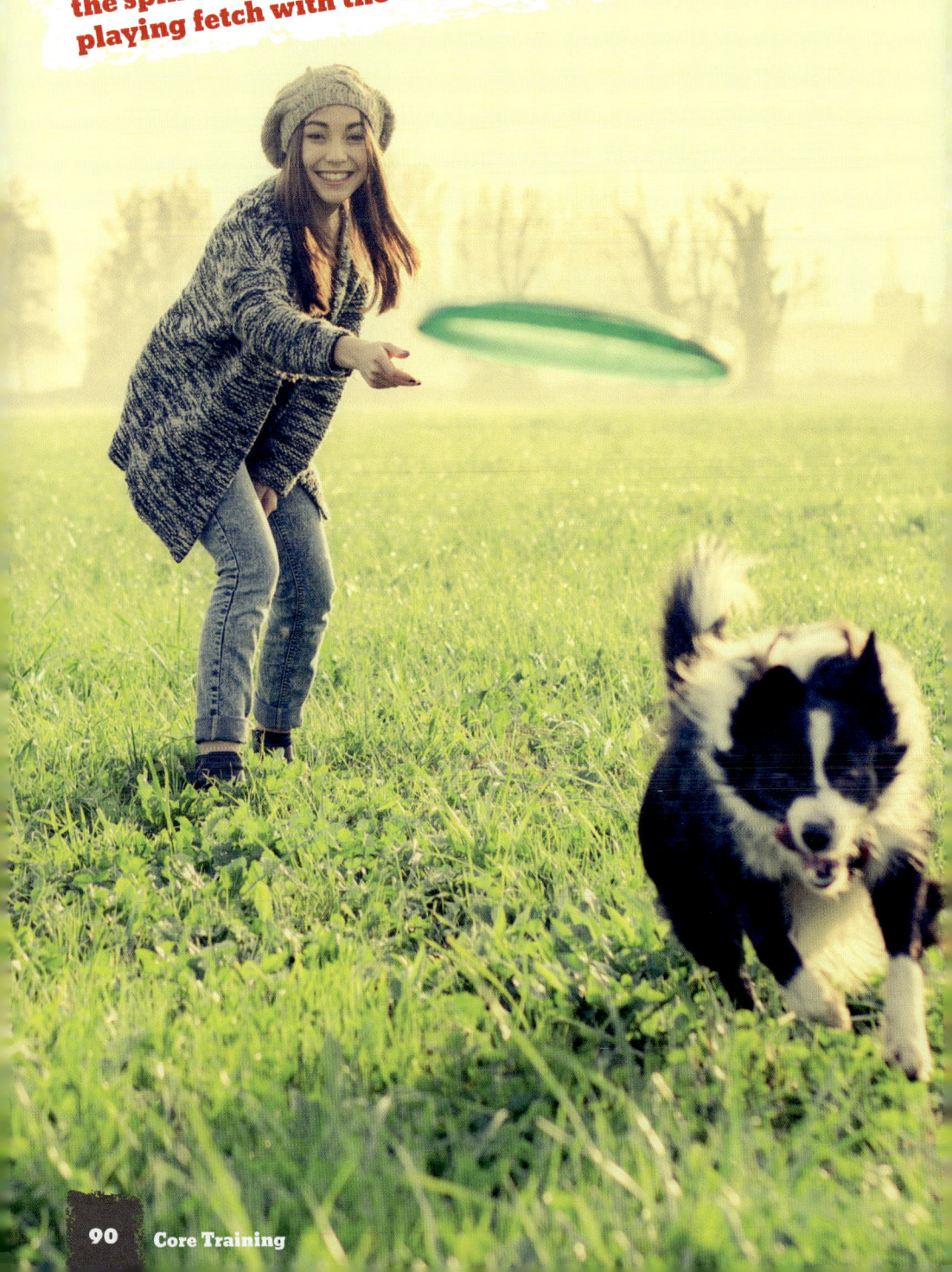

Exercises that help to control excessive upper body movement can help to protect the spine during everyday activities like playing fetch with the dog.